# LIVING THE
# MEDITERRANEAN DIET

## PROVEN PRINCIPLES & MODERN RECIPES FOR STAYING HEALTHY

Nick Nigro & Bay Ewald
with Rea Frey

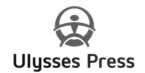

**Ulysses Press**

Published in the U.S. by
Ulysses Press
P.O. Box 3440
Berkeley, CA 94703
www.ulyssespress.com

ISBN: 978-1-61243-431-5
Library of Congress Control Number 2014952010

Printed in Korea by WE SP through Four Colour Print Group

10 9 8 7 6 5 4 3 2 1

Acquisitions editor: Keith Riegert
Managing editor: Claire Chun
Editor: Alice Riegert
Copyeditor: Lauren Harrison
Proofreader: Renee Rutledge
Cover and interior design: Ashley Prine
Layout and production: Jake Flaherty
Index: Sayre Van Young
Interior photographs: © Nick Nigro and Bay Ewald except on pages 28–29, 31, 37, 49, 50, 125, 130, 133 (except bottom right) © Dulcet Creative; pages 76–77, 92, 101 © Meiwen Wang
Cover photographs: © Nick Nigro and Bay Ewald except top row front © Dulcet Creative, beets © Meiwen Wang

Distributed by Publishers Group West

IMPORTANT NOTE TO READERS: This book has been written and published strictly for informational and educational purposes only. It is not intended to serve as medical advice or to be any form of medical treatment. You should always consult your physician before altering or changing any aspect of your medical treatment and/or undertaking a diet regimen, including the guidelines as described in this book. Do not stop or change any prescription medications without the guidance and advice of your physician. Any use of the information in this book is made on the reader's good judgment after consulting with his or her physician and is the reader's sole responsibility. This book is not intended to diagnose or treat any medical condition and is not a substitute for a physician.

This book is independently authored and published and no sponsorship or endorsement of this book by, and no affiliation with, any trademarked brands or other products mentioned within is claimed or suggested. All trademarks that appear in this book belong to their respective owners and are used here for informational purposes only. The author and publishers encourage readers to patronize the quality brands and products mentioned in this book.

*We dedicate this cookbook to Gloria Bos—Gram.*
*We thank you for sharing your kitchen and your wisdom.*
*And to Carter Dean Smith—may your curiosity always inspire you to create and dream.*
*We love you both.*

# CONTENTS

INTRODUCTION . . . . . . . . . . . . . . . . . . . . . . . . . . . . . . . . . . . . . . . . . . . . . . . . . . . . . . 8

THE MEDITERRANEAN DIET . . . . . . . . . . . . . . . . . . . . . . . . . . . . . . . . . . . 11

## SPRING . . . . . . . . . . . . . . . . . . . . . . . . . . . . . . . . . . . . . . . . . . . . 29

Watermelon Gazpacho . . . . . . . . . . . . . . . . . . . . . . . . . . . . . . . . . . . . . . . . 30

Asparagus, Prosciutto, and Mushroom Pizza . . . . . . . . . . . . . . . . . . . . . . . . . 32

Black Peppered Lamb Chops with Mint-Yogurt Sauce . . . . . . . . . . . . . . . . . . 34

Farfalle Pasta with Arugula, Tomatoes, and Sunflower Seed Pesto . . . . . . . . . 36

Mediterranean Chicken Stir-Fry . . . . . . . . . . . . . . . . . . . . . . . . . . . . . . . . . . 38

Broccoli Pecan Ravioli . . . . . . . . . . . . . . . . . . . . . . . . . . . . . . . . . . . . . . . . . 39

Tuna Steaks with Caper, Olive, and Sun-Dried Tomato Relish . . . . . . . . . . . . . 40

Caesar Salad with Mesquite Grilled Chicken and Homemade Dressing . . . . . . . 42

Roasted Veggie Tower . . . . . . . . . . . . . . . . . . . . . . . . . . . . . . . . . . . . . . . . . 44

Balsamic-Marinated Portobello Mushrooms . . . . . . . . . . . . . . . . . . . . . . . . . 45

Mediterranean Rice Salad . . . . . . . . . . . . . . . . . . . . . . . . . . . . . . . . . . . . . . 46

Swiss Chard Chardonnay Sauté . . . . . . . . . . . . . . . . . . . . . . . . . . . . . . . . . . 47

Lemon-Thyme Sorbet in Lemon Cups . . . . . . . . . . . . . . . . . . . . . . . . . . . . . . 48

Grapefruit Mint Prosecco . . . . . . . . . . . . . . . . . . . . . . . . . . . . . . . . . . . . . . 51

## SUMMER . . . . . . . . . . . . . . . . . . . . . . . . . . . . . . . . . . . . . . . . . . . 53

Caprese Boats . . . . . . . . . . . . . . . . . . . . . . . . . . . . . . . . . . . . . . . . . . . . . . 54

Chilled Avocado-Cucumber Soup . . . . . . . . . . . . . . . . . . . . . . . . . . . . . . . . . 55

Cucumber Salad with Crumbled Feta and Pine Nuts . . . . . . . . . . . . . . . . . . . . 56

Grilled Prosciutto e Melone . . . . . . . . . . . . . . . . . . . . . . . . . . . . . . . . . . . . . 58

Avocado and Lime Shrimp Cocktail . . . . . . . . . . . . . . . . . . . . . . . . . . . . . . . . 60

Wild Salmon on Pecan Wood with Dill-Yogurt Sauce . . . . . . . . . . . . . . . . . . . 62

Orange and Fennel Salad with White Wine Citrus Dressing . . . . . . . . . . . . . . . 64

Almond Baked Halibut with Tomato-Caper Sauce . . . . . . . . . . . . . . . . . . . . . . 65

Eggplant and Kalamata Rolls. . . . . . . . . . . . . . . . . . . . . . . . . . . . . . . . . . . . . . . . 66

Mediterranean Ceviche . . . . . . . . . . . . . . . . . . . . . . . . . . . . . . . . . . . . . . . . . . . . 67

Heirloom Tomato and Kale Pizza with Herb Pizza Dough . . . . . . . . . . . . . . . . 68

Garlic-Herb Rice . . . . . . . . . . . . . . . . . . . . . . . . . . . . . . . . . . . . . . . . . . . . . . . . . . 70

Spearmint-Pistachio Gelato . . . . . . . . . . . . . . . . . . . . . . . . . . . . . . . . . . . . . . . . 71

Mascarpone and Honey Stuffed Figs with a Balsamic Reduction . . . . . . . . . . . 72

Honey-Fig Jam . . . . . . . . . . . . . . . . . . . . . . . . . . . . . . . . . . . . . . . . . . . . . . . . . . . 74

## AUTUMN . . . . . . . . . . . . . . . . . . . . . . . . . . . . . . . 77

Avocado Deviled Eggs . . . . . . . . . . . . . . . . . . . . . . . . . . . . . . . . . . . . . . . . . . . . . 78

Butternut Squash–Pomegranate Hummus . . . . . . . . . . . . . . . . . . . . . . . . . . . . 81

Red Wine and Garlic Steamed Mussels . . . . . . . . . . . . . . . . . . . . . . . . . . . . . . . 82

Zucchini Lasagna . . . . . . . . . . . . . . . . . . . . . . . . . . . . . . . . . . . . . . . . . . . . . . . . . 85

Barley Risotto with Mushroom, Fig, and Arugula . . . . . . . . . . . . . . . . . . . . . . . 87

Garlic-Herb Spaghetti Squash with Lemon . . . . . . . . . . . . . . . . . . . . . . . . . . . . 88

Sweet Potato Gnocchi with Honey Crisp Apples . . . . . . . . . . . . . . . . . . . . . . . . 90

Beet Carpaccio. . . . . . . . . . . . . . . . . . . . . . . . . . . . . . . . . . . . . . . . . . . . . . . . . . . 93

Whole Roasted Apple-Rosemary Chicken . . . . . . . . . . . . . . . . . . . . . . . . . . . . . 94

Pear and Prosecco Tilapia . . . . . . . . . . . . . . . . . . . . . . . . . . . . . . . . . . . . . . . . . . 95

Simple Sautéed Rapini . . . . . . . . . . . . . . . . . . . . . . . . . . . . . . . . . . . . . . . . . . . . 96

Mint-Carrot Cabbage Wedge . . . . . . . . . . . . . . . . . . . . . . . . . . . . . . . . . . . . . . . 97

Baked Lemon and Thyme Mushrooms . . . . . . . . . . . . . . . . . . . . . . . . . . . . . . . . 98

Roasted Pumpkin Apple Sage Soup. . . . . . . . . . . . . . . . . . . . . . . . . . . . . . . . . 100

Almond Flour Zucchini-Carrot Breakfast Cake. . . . . . . . . . . . . . . . . . . . . . . . . 103

## WINTER. . . . . . . . . . . . . . . . . . . . . . . . . . . . . . . . 105

Warm Rosemary Olives. . . . . . . . . . . . . . . . . . . . . . . . . . . . . . . . . . . . . . . . . . . 106

Tuscan Tomato and Cannellini Bean Soup with Kale. . . . . . . . . . . . . . . . . . . . 107

Roasted Fennel and Cauliflower Soup . . . . . . . . . . . . . . . . . . . . . . . . . . . . . . . 109

Cioppino . . . . . . . . . . . . . . . . . . . . . . . . . . . . . . . . . . . . . . . . . . . . . . . . . . . . . . . 110

Spaghetti and Turkey Meatballs. . . . . . . . . . . . . . . . . . . . . . . . . . . . . . . . . . . . 112

Chicken Sausage Barley Risotto with Rapini and Sun-Dried Tomatoes . . . . . . 114

Seared Scallops over Spinach . . . . . . . . . . . . . . . . . . . . . . . . . . . . . . . . . . . . . . 116

Peppered Swordfish with Warm Chive-Garlic Sauce . . . . . . . . . . . . . . . . . . . . . . . . . . . . 117

Linguine and Clam Sauce . . . . . . . . . . . . . . . . . . . . . . . . . . . . . . . . . . . . . . . . . . . . . . . 118

Beef Braciole . . . . . . . . . . . . . . . . . . . . . . . . . . . . . . . . . . . . . . . . . . . . . . . . . . . . . . . . 120

Winter Chicory with Persimmons . . . . . . . . . . . . . . . . . . . . . . . . . . . . . . . . . . . . . . . . . 122

Quinoa Kale Salad with Roasted Butternut Squash . . . . . . . . . . . . . . . . . . . . . . . . . . 125

Roasted Mediterranean Brussels Sprouts . . . . . . . . . . . . . . . . . . . . . . . . . . . . . . . . . . 126

Chicken Piccata . . . . . . . . . . . . . . . . . . . . . . . . . . . . . . . . . . . . . . . . . . . . . . . . . . . . . . . 128

Dark Chocolate Tangerine Slices . . . . . . . . . . . . . . . . . . . . . . . . . . . . . . . . . . . . . . . . . 129

# APPENDIX . . . . . . . . . . . . . . . . . . . . . . . . . . . . . 130

Fresh Pasta Dough . . . . . . . . . . . . . . . . . . . . . . . . . . . . . . . . . . . . . . . . . . . . . . . . . . . 131

Fresh Pizza Dough . . . . . . . . . . . . . . . . . . . . . . . . . . . . . . . . . . . . . . . . . . . . . . . . . . . 134

Sample Menus for Every-days and Extraordinary-days . . . . . . . . . . . . . . . . . . . . . . 135

# REFERENCES . . . . . . . . . . . . . . . . . . . . . . . . . . . . . . . . . . . . . . . . . . . . . . . . . . . . . 138

# CONVERSIONS . . . . . . . . . . . . . . . . . . . . . . . . . . . . . . . . . . . . . . . . . . . . . . . . . . . 138

# INDEX . . . . . . . . . . . . . . . . . . . . . . . . . . . . . . . . . . . . . . . . . . . . . . . . . . . . . . . . . . . 140

# ACKNOWLEDGMENTS . . . . . . . . . . . . . . . . . . . . . . . . . . . . . . . . . . . . . . . . . . . . . 143

# ABOUT THE AUTHORS . . . . . . . . . . . . . . . . . . . . . . . . . . . . . . . . . . . . . . . . . . . . 144

# INTRODUCTION

We met on a cold evening a few days after Christmas in San Francisco. Bundled up in beanies and sweaters with our good friends, we ventured to Scoma's in Fisherman's Wharf, a bustling yet intimate place on the water. From there, as we munched on calamari and broiled wild king salmon, it became love at first meal. We spent the next 30 days straight together, adventuring up and down the California coast, eating, laughing, and falling deeper into a food-filled romance. When Nick made his way back to Orange County and Bay stayed in San Francisco to finish graduate school, nightly conversations often, if not always, revolved around our grandiose dreams and big plans once we were able to finally live in the same city.

In October 2013, we launched comewecreate, a boutique culinary arts company that focuses on all creative aspects of food through design, photography, written words, film and recipe development. We see food as the fundamental building block to all of our endeavors—the thing that helps us make sense out of our crazy, hectic, bizarrely beautiful life together. Whatever has gone on in our days, whether individually or together, we come to the kitchen to put on our favorite tunes, light a candle, and reconnect with ourselves and with each other.

We both come from families who cooked healthy and wholesome meals, and when we moved in together, the idea of a Mediterranean diet wasn't something we plotted or planned—it was just the way we instinctively ate. Nick grew up in an Italian-American family with traditions and recipes that had been passed on for generations, and Bay grew up on an avocado farm in a rural area where nearly every meal was homemade.

Over the years, we began to notice that on days when we filled our bodies with whole grains, fresh fish, and beautiful plant-based foods, we felt good. We had more energy, more patience, and were more lively. We had those days, of course, when we indulged in one too many treats or french fries, but we made sure to remember how good we felt when we were eating the Mediterranean way, and that always encouraged us to get back on track.

What we hope is that the Mediterranean lifestyle—and this book—can give you what it has given us: the ability to feel good from the inside out. Our diet is one of abundance, not restriction, a combination of tastes with healthy foods full of vibrant colors and rich aromas, traditional recipes with modern twists that will transport you across the Atlantic Ocean. We want to emphasize the importance of enjoying your meals and an active life with those you love, to trust your instincts, heart, and mind in the kitchen and in life, to taste, see, feel, and hear every bit of the world around you. We want you to love—to really love—the life you lead and the food that nourishes that life.

May you bring your own soul and your own piece of you into the recipes that follow.

*Mangia bene*—Eat well!

—Nick and Bay

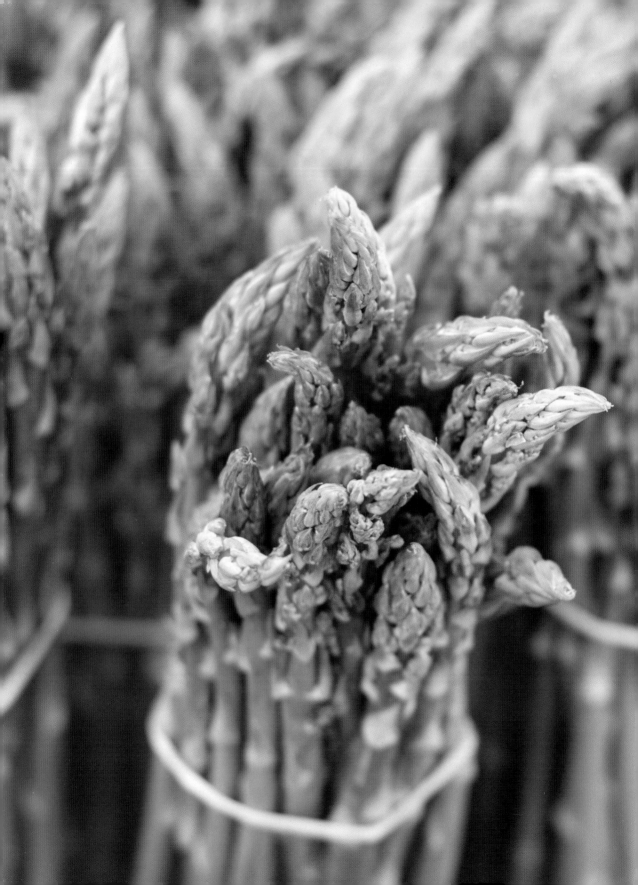

# THE MEDITERRANEAN DIET

Before delving into the recipes, let's take a look at what comprises the Mediterranean diet. It revolves around healthier, sustainable principles of eating and living. It's not a "diet" in a traditional sense—it's a lifestyle.

The Mediterranean diet is a plant-based diet consisting of eating whole, unprocessed foods, such as vegetables and fruits, as well as whole grains, good fats from nuts, seeds, and olive oil, and fresh seafood. These are the *staple* foods of a Mediterranean diet, though good-quality dairy, meat, and poultry make appearances as well. Because this diet is primarily plant-based, you will effortlessly increase the amount of fruits and veggies you eat, which improves fiber intake and the overall quality of your nutrition.

Mediterranean eating stems from southern Italy, Greece, Spain, and Morocco. Traditionally, people ate fresh, whole foods instead of the processed fare of today. They caught fish from the sea, enjoyed unaltered whole grains, fruits, vegetables, and delicious fats from olives and olive oil.

The roots of a Mediterranean diet are rich. It's not just about food—there's a *lifestyle* attached. It's about eating with your family and enjoying your food. It's about being active. It's about food making you healthy *and* happy. It's about balance. It's about slowing our manic pace to a reasonable jaunt.

History is a strange beast. While milk and meat gained traction in the 1940s, the Mediterranean people sat, indifferent, eating the way their ancestors had. In Marissa Cloutier and Eve Adamson's book, *The Mediterranean Diet*, they discuss a thorough investigation of the way Mediterranean people ate. Conducted by the Rockefeller Foundation in 1948, a study by epidemiologist Leland Allbaugh found that this Cretan diet "derived approximately 61 percent of its calories from plant foods, only 7 percent from animal foods, and a full 38 percent of total calories from fat." The findings? This way of eating was *very* conducive to heart health. While everyone jumped on the meat and dairy bandwagon, the Mediterranean people stuck true to what they knew and loved. They thrived and prospered and maintained their health.

Throughout time, waves of dietary change have come and gone: low-fat, nonfat, low-carb, high-carb, vegan, Paleo, etc. These diets are marketed with the promise to promote health and happiness, but they are usually entrenched with all-or-nothing claims, gimmicks, and short-lived dietary plans that are not enjoyable or sustainable. They simply don't (and can't) last.

The Mediterranean diet works. It's easy. There's no deprivation of any food group. There are recommended *restrictions* of certain foods that aren't beneficial to health, but there are ample choices to maintain variety and satiety for all palettes. Research consistently proves that eating a heart-healthy Mediterranean diet will slash cancer and stroke risks, eradicate preventable diseases, and boost the *quality* of life—not just your quantity of years.

# THE SAD TRUTH

It's no surprise that when following a Mediterranean diet, which promotes healthy fats, produce, whole grains, and seafood, you have lower risks of heart disease and cholesterol, have lower body mass indexes, and experience more heart-healthy benefits. By sticking to healthy portions of fresh food in its natural state, you will obtain all the nutrients needed to nourish the body.

But how can a diet rich in fat be healthier than what average Americans eat? Because those fats don't come from animals. Americans consume *saturated* fat, which hinders health. Saturated fats raise cholesterol and can contribute to heart disease. People of the Mediterranean eat *monounsaturated* fat from plant sources, which promotes heart health. Monounsaturated fats lower cholesterol and reduce the risks of heart disease and stroke. Marissa Cloutier and Eve Adamson note in *The Mediterranean Diet* that "according to researcher Ancel Keys, Cretans consumed about ½ cup of olive oil per day, per person! Heart disease rates in the southern, or rather the Mediterranean, regions of Italy, Spain, and France were also remarkably low." It's not always about calories, fat, or protein. It's about the *source* of our food and the *quality* of our ingredients.

With *Living the Mediterranean Diet*, there's nothing "added" to the staples of these dishes, such as the trans fat, salt, and sugar that most Americans consume on a meal-by-meal basis. The average American is now experiencing regular obesity and sickness, with heart disease as the number one killer of men and women. Americans are so stressed that chowing down on fast food and melting into the couch at the end of an interminably long day has become the norm.

America as a whole has gone from eating natural foods and moving for our professions (physical labor) to a "convenient" diet, full of processed foods and produce packed with chemicals and pesticides, and living completely sedentary lifestyles. Think about our culture: We are hyperfocused on the concept of living to work instead of working to live. Americans have grown increasingly more stressed, less healthy, and more constrained with every decade that passes. In Angelo Acquista's book, *The Mediterranean Prescription*, he reveals that "approximately two out of three Americans are either overweight or obese (compared with fewer than one out of four in the early 1960s), and that obesity may shorten life span by five to twenty years." While many of us know that heart disease, cancer, and stroke are the leading causes of death, what we might not know is that these causes "are all exacerbated or caused by excess weight." It's time to make a change.

# THE PRINCIPLES OF THE MEDITERRANEAN DIET

*Living the Mediterranean Diet* addresses our *current* daily concerns and makes every choice easier. If you consciously pick natural foods as the staple of your meals, you will be successful. If you decide that you are going to enjoy dinner with your family, you will be successful. If you decide that laughter is more important than stress, you will be successful.

Though we will break down exactly what foods one eats on a Mediterranean diet on the pages that follow, let's look at what makes up the basics of nutrition.

# MACRONUTRIENTS

Macronutrients are essential for us to grow. They consist of fats, proteins, carbohydrates, and water. We need macronutrients in decent doses to survive.

**FATS:** Fats are a wonderful fuel source and provide essential fatty acids, which help our brains function properly and curbs inflammation.

**PROTEINS:** Proteins help repair the body and promote muscle growth.

**CARBOHYDRATES:** Carbohydrates act as a primary fuel source. They are our energy.

**WATER:** Water helps us stay hydrated, regulates body temperature, and flushes toxins from the system.

# MICRONUTRIENTS

Micronutrients are needed in much smaller doses than macronutrients are. They are composed of vitamins and minerals, and are essential to help us with metabolic processes and protect us from diseases.

**VITAMINS:** Vitamins are found in fruits and vegetables and help promote health. Vitamins include A, B, biotin, C, choline, D, E, folic acid, and K.

**MINERALS:** Minerals are inorganic substances that come from the soil or water and help the body build bones and strong teeth, and they aid in muscle contractions, blood clotting, enzyme regulation, and more. Minerals include calcium, chloride, chromium, copper, fluoride, iodine, iron, magnesium, manganese, phosphorous, potassium, sodium, sulfur, and zinc.

# THE MAINSTAY OF THE MEDITERRANEAN DIET

Because the mainstay of a Mediterranean diet covers both macro- and micronutrients, focus on the following three choices as the *mainstay* of your diet to reap the most nutritional benefits.

**PRODUCE:** Full of antioxidants (which help protect cells against damage from free radicals), vitamins, phytonutrients, and minerals, think of all fruits and vegetables as your cancer fighters, because they stave off disease and arm the body with nutrients to fight off invaders. Produce should make up the bulk of your dietary choices on the Mediterranean diet.

**WHOLE GRAINS:** Loaded with fiber and other nutrients, whole grains act as preventatives to stomach issues and insulin spikes. Think of grains as the disease prevention of your diet. They also provide fuel for daily activities. Whole grains are a large component of the Mediterranean diet and should be eaten daily.

**FATS:** Do not fear fat! Fats from good sources, such as oily fish, nuts, seeds, and extra-virgin olive oil, reduce inflammation in the body, protect the joints, and can even give the skin a radiant boost. Fats are your protectors.

# THE NUTRITIONAL BREAKDOWN

While there are no hard and fast rules for *Living the Mediterranean Diet*, it's imperative to make daily choices that will result in optimal health. On the pages that follow, you'll find guidelines to help you on your way. In terms of food, stick to *organic* produce and *wild* fish whenever possible. Think about where your food is coming from and how many ingredients it contains.

In America, we have a skewed vision of what we think proper portion sizes are. Take an Italian restaurant for example. We could eat up to 6 or 7 cups of pasta, when a proper portion size is just ½ cup! Once you get used to measuring out proper ½ cup to 1 cup portions, you will be able to eyeball what a proper portion size should be. Make sure to load up the majority of your plate with fresh veggies, and if eating meat, reduce to the size of a deck of cards. No 20-ounce sirloins allowed. Proper portions for the foods included on the diet are as follows:

| FOOD | RECOMMENDED SERVINGS | SERVING SIZE |
|------|---------------------|--------------|
| Whole grains | 4 to 6 per day | ½ cup cooked grains like oats, quinoa, or pasta, or 1 slice of bread |
| Vegetables | 4 to 8 per day | 1 cup raw vegetables or ½ cup cooked vegetables |
| Fruits | 2 to 4 per day | ½ cup fresh fruit (or 1 average piece of fruit) or ¼ cup dried fruit |
| Beans and legumes | 1 to 3 per day | ⅓ cup dried beans or 1 cup cooked beans |
| Seafood | 2 to 3 servings per week | 4 to 6 ounces |
| Fats | 3 to 6 per day | 1 ounce nuts or seeds (this can range anywhere from 12 to 40 nuts, depending on the size) or 2 tablespoons ground nut and seed butters; for oils, a serving size is usually 1 tablespoon |
| Herbs/spices/ condiments | | For condiments, aim for 1 tablespoon; fresh or dried herbs can be used in unlimited quantities; salt should be reduced to 1 to 2 teaspoons per day. |

| FOOD | RECOMMENDED SERVINGS | SERVING SIZE |
|---|---|---|
| Poultry | 1 to 3 servings per week | 3 to 4 ounces (it should fit in the palm of your hand) |
| Red meat | 3 to 4 times per month | 3 ounces |
| Eggs | 3 to 4 times per week (egg whites can be eaten daily) | 1 egg |
| Dairy | 1 to 3 per day | 1 cup yogurt or 1 ounce cheese |
| Alcohol | Aim for no more than one drink per day | A serving size of alcohol is 4 ounces of wine or 12 ounces of beer. |
| Sweets | Avoid | Opt for one serving of fruit in lieu of other sugars |

## WHOLE GRAINS

Grains are full of nutrients, fiber, protein, and those ever-important complex carbohydrates that supply energy. In Western diets, carbohydrates often get a bad rap, but they are vital to providing nutrients and supplying our bodies with energy. They also help the body feel satiated. When choosing grains, make sure they have not been refined in any way. Refined grains, such as white bread and pasta, have little nutritional value. These grains have been stripped of important nutrients, and synthetic vitamins and minerals are added back in. Because they lack fiber, they will raise insulin levels as well. Whole grains, on the other hand, contain fiber, which keeps blood sugar stable. Whole grains also keep you full, which prevents overeating. Choose from popular Mediterranean grains such as amaranth, barley, black rice, brown rice, buckwheat, bulgur, couscous, emmer, farro, jasmine rice, Kamut, kasha, millet, oats, oat groats, polenta, potatoes, quinoa, red clover, red rice, rye, spelt, wheat, wheat berries, and wild rice.

## VEGETABLES

Vegetables are bright colored for a reason. They contain flavonoids, carotenoids, and chlorophyll, which give veggies their different hues. In addition, veggies contain phytonutrients, which are natural chemicals that help protect plants from germs. Phytonutrients also help your body work at peak levels and promote overall health. When selecting vegetables, choose from the colors of the rainbow to ensure you're getting a good assortment of vitamins and minerals. Vitamins and minerals are essential to ensuring proper bodily functions and must be ingested from outside sources (meaning our bodies don't make them on their own). Getting vitamins and minerals from whole foods, such as produce, rather than synthetic vitamins, such as store-bought vitamins or manufactured varieties added into processed foods, makes a huge difference in how our bodies absorb them. Our bodies absorb vitamins and minerals most efficiently when they come from real food.

When choosing vegetables, think green (potassium and vitamin K), yellow (lutein and vitamin C), red (lycopene and folate), orange (vitamin C and omegas), and purple (vitamin A, vitamin B2, and iron). Don't just reach for the same old potatoes or corn. Sample options to include in the Mediterranean diet include: artichokes, arugula, asparagus, beets, broccoli, brussels sprouts, carrots, cauliflower, celery, chives, collard greens, cucumber, eggplant, fennel, kale, leeks, mushrooms, onions, parsnips, peppers, pumpkin, rapini, romaine, Swiss chard, turnip greens, and squash.

# EAT YOUR PRODUCE

Because this diet is hyperfocused on getting fruits and vegetables into your diet, follow these tips for eating more produce.

DRINK SMOOTHIES. A great go-to for those who don't love their veggies, simply blend up two fruits of your choice, a handful of greens, such as kale and spinach, and some parsley or cilantro, and enjoy a delicious green shake with nearly half your daily intake of fruits and veggies in one fell swoop. It's a great, nutritious way to start your morning.

MAKE VEGGIES THE STAR. When eating lunch or dinner, think about vegetables as the star and your protein as a side dish. The recipes in this book are a great example of how to change your mentality to let the produce shine.

PICK ONE COLOR PER MEAL. If you get overwhelmed or often waste produce because you buy too much and then it sits at the back of your fridge, untouched, focus on one color of the rainbow and plan your meals around that. If you pick red, for instance, perhaps enjoy a beet and apple smoothie at breakfast, a delicious tomato salad at lunch and salmon and red potatoes at dinner. Think simple.

EAT MONO MEALS. When it comes to fruits and veggies, simple is often the way to go. Eating a handful of berries or grilling up some zucchini drizzled in olive oil can be a satisfying way to curb hunger and get an extra dose of produce in your day.

PAIR WITH A PROTEIN. Any time you're going to eat a protein, such as fish or meat, pair it with some greens. Make this a staple for lunch or dinner and you'll meet your daily quota in no time.

## FRUITS

Full of easy-to-digest fiber and sugars that won't elicit an insulin response, fruit is one of the most perfect foods, full of bold flavors. Fruit is best eaten on an empty stomach. It's made to pass through the body quickly, and if eaten after other foods (or even mixed with heavier foods, such as proteins), it gets "stuck" in the gut and can putrefy. Some fruits have a lot of sugar, but because fruit contains soluble fiber, which acts as a "natural blood sugar blocker," it doesn't cause an insulin response like added sugars in most processed foods or desserts do. Choose from apples, apricots, avocado, bananas, blackberries, blueberries, boysenberries, cantaloupe, cherries, dates, figs, grapes, grapefruit, guava, kumquats, lemons, limes, nectarines, olives, oranges, peaches, pears, pineapples, plums, pomegranates, tomatoes, and watermelon. Have a dessert craving? Opt for fresh fruit whenever possible.

## BEANS AND LEGUMES

Beans and legumes are one of the most perfect foods around. With just 1 cup, you receive 16 to 28 grams of protein, as well as fiber, iron, B vitamins, and minerals. Another perk? They're more affordable than meat-based proteins. It's recommended that you buy dry beans whenever possible, as canning reduces nutrients. Simply soak them in water overnight and cook the next day after rinsing thoroughly. (Lentils and peanuts do not need to be soaked.) This will cut down on the cooking time and help rid the legumes of phytates, acids that make them difficult to digest.

---

# THE IMPORTANCE OF FIBER

Fiber helps keep us fuller longer and tames cravings. It allows our systems to stay regular by facilitating proper elimination (i.e., pushing waste out). All plant foods contain soluble fiber (which dissolves in water) or insoluble fiber (which does not dissolve in water). Soluble fiber swells when mixed with water, which helps keep blood glucose levels stable by providing a slow and constant stream of glucose instead of an immediate release of sugar to your liver. Good sources of soluble fiber include fruits, veggies, and legumes. Insoluble fiber does not break down and often passes through the body in its original form. Because it doesn't break down, it can help ease constipation and keep our systems regular by pushing along other foods in the digestive tract. While certain fruits and veggies contain insoluble fiber, whole grains are its primary sources.

When aiming to get enough fiber in the diet, eat a wide variety of fruits, vegetables, whole grains, nuts, and seeds—which also happen to be the high-quality staple foods of a Mediterranean diet! The average American does not consume enough fiber, getting only around 10 to 15 grams per day. We should aim to get 25 to 35 grams per day and drink plenty of water to keep our bodies functioning optimally.

---

Choose from adzuki, black, cannellini, chickpeas, cranberry beans, fava, great northern, kidney, lentils, lima, mung, navy, peanuts, peas, pinto, and split peas.

## SEAFOOD

Seafood contains a host of heart-healthy nutrients. When opting for fish, choose from oilier varieties, such as salmon, trout, mackerel, herring, and sardines. The oilier the fish, the more heart-healthy fats it contains. Fish are one of the best sources of omega-3 fatty acids, which the body cannot produce on its own. These fats help the brain function and act as inflammation fighters in the body. Besides these important fats, fish and seafood are a wonderful source of protein. Per ounce, fish contains around 6 grams of protein, while red meat and chicken contain around 7 grams per ounce and pork contains around 6 grams per ounce. Love seafood? Choose from high-quality sources, such as scallops, shrimp, mussels, and crab, which are high in vitamins and minerals and can be a wonderful addition to any meal. Worried about mercury? Do your homework to see where your fish is coming from and choose from the freshest, most sustainable selections available.

Good sources include albacore tuna, clams, cod, crab, flounder, haddock, halibut, herring, lobsters, mussels, pollock, salmon, sardines, scallops, shrimp, snapper, squid, and trout.

## FATS

Fats are crucial to proper bodily functions. They provide essential fatty acids that cannot be manufactured in the body. Fats can also prevent inflammatory responses in the body and lower

---

# THE SKINNY ON FAT

When deciding what fats to consume, make sure you understand what's considered "healthy" and what isn't. To put it simply, monounsaturated and polyunsaturated fats are good. Saturated fats and trans fats are bad. Typically, we want to avoid foods high in cholesterol as well. Fatty meats, trans fats, dairy products, and egg yolks are all high in cholesterol and should be consumed in moderation or avoided altogether. Choose from the healthy fats list when making smart dietary choices.

### HEALTHY FATS

Monounsaturated fats: olive oil, nuts, seeds, and avocados

Polyunsaturated fats (omega-3 and -6): nuts, seeds, and fatty fish

### UNHEALTHY FATS

Saturated fats: red meat, dairy, and butter

Trans fats: processed foods and foods containing hydrogenated or partially hydrogenated oils

our risk for chronic diseases. However, there are good fats and bad fats, and we are often confused about how much we should get and from what sources. Choose from foods that are in their most natural state and provide more than just fat. Most raw nuts and seeds, peanuts, avocados, olives, and of course, extra-virgin olive oil, are important dietary staples for a good Mediterranean diet. Make sure you purchase quality olive oil. In recent years, scams have

## THE DIRTY DOZEN AND THE CLEAN FIFTEEN

The Environmental Working Group put together the latest list of the top 51 foods that were dirtiest to cleanest, as well as an updated version of the "dirty dozen" and the "clean fifteen." The dirty dozen, which are conventional fruits and veggies, were found to contain at least 47 different chemicals. When purchasing the produce on the dirty dozen list, always opt for organic; avoid them altogether if organic isn't an option.

### DIRTY DOZEN

* Apples
* Celery
* Cherry tomatoes
* Cucumbers
* Grapes
* Nectarines (imported)
* Peaches
* Potatoes
* Snap peas (imported)
* Spinach
* Strawberries
* Sweet bell peppers

If you can't afford organic produce, the "clean fifteen" contain lower to no traces of pesticides and are considered safe to consume in conventional form.

### CLEAN FIFTEEN

* Asparagus
* Avocados
* Cabbage
* Cantaloupe
* Cauliflower
* Eggplant
* Grapefruit
* Kiwis
* Mangos
* Onions
* Papayas
* Pineapples
* Sweet corn
* Sweet peas (frozen)
* Sweet potatoes

surfaced where distributors are replacing olive oil with cheap ingredients. See olive oil on sale for a price that's too good to be true? It probably is! Purchase brands you trust.

## HERBS, SPICES, AND CONDIMENTS

Herbs and spices can take a boring dish and make it amazing, all without adding extra fat or salt. Experiment with flavors to see what your palate enjoys and don't be afraid to vary it often. There is a wide variety of Greek favorites, but balsamic vinegar, basil, bay leaves, capers, cayenne, cilantro, cinnamon, garlic, oregano, paprika, parsley, peppers, rosemary, saffron, (high-quality) salt, sumac, turmeric, thyme, vinegar, and za'atar add zest and succulent flavor to a magnitude of dishes. The best thing about herbs and spices is that they're medicinal. They contain antioxidants, can curb inflammation, are antiviral, antifungal, and antimicrobial, can ease digestive disorders, increase circulation, and can even alleviate nausea. Diets high in herbs and spices can act as preventatives from common colds and flus and help the body function optimally.

## POULTRY, RED MEAT, AND EGGS

Poultry, red meat, and eggs have been staples of the American diet for quite some time. They are good sources of protein, but the amounts we eat have become a problem over the years. From factory farming to hormone-injected and antibiotic-fed poultry and meat, these "staples" have caused more harm than good in recent years. While eggs can be a great source of protein, the yolks are high in cholesterol and should be limited to four times per week. Always opt for organic, humane-certified eggs whenever possible. In addition, the amount of red meat we eat has been linked to higher rates of heart disease. From the way red meat and poultry is cooked to the treatment of factory-farmed animals, there are many reasons to cut back on it. Not only are meat and poultry more expensive than plant-based foods, they are harder to digest and very acidic in the body. Try and cut back on meat and poultry, and choose from organic local options or grass-fed whenever possible. Typical meats in a Mediterranean diet include chicken, goat, lamb, pork, veal, and wild rabbit. Eggs are also a staple.

## DAIRY

Dairy comes in many forms: milk, cream, yogurt, and cheese. These products come in nonfat, low-fat, or full-fat options. Whenever possible, choose the unaltered, full-fat version. When food is nonfat or low-fat, it has been processed. The fat is stripped away and synthetic chemicals, additives, vitamins, and extra sugars are often put back in. Dairy can also be extremely acidic and hard to digest. Opting for sheep's or goat's cheese or milk, which is easier to digest than cow's milk, can be a great alternative to traditional dairy. While cheese is used in many dishes in the Mediterranean diet, it's consumed in moderation. Because we can't often get the same quality and freshness of cheese in the States as in Greece, always search for the highest quality of ingredients (no Velveeta!). Opt for goat's cheese, sheep's milk cheese (such as feta, Manchego,

Manouri, Pecorino, and ricotta), blue cheese, brie, cheddar, cottage cheese, plain Greek yogurt, mozzarella, Parmigiano-Reggiano, and Swiss.

## OTHER

While red wine has many heart-health benefits, it's still alcohol and is high in sugar, so drink it in moderation. The same goes for sweets. If you love chocolate, opt for dark varieties for the most antioxidants. Make smart choices and indulge sparingly!

# THE LIFESTYLE

As we mentioned, *Living the Mediterranean Diet* isn't just about food. To partake in the Mediterranean diet means that you are *choosing* to live a certain lifestyle. You're not just making better food choices—you're making better choices, period. You're laughing more, enjoying life more, slowing down, working smarter not harder, being more active, and staying in tune with who you really are and what you really want.

That's what *Living the Mediterranean Diet* is. We live in *modern* times that are different, times that move at lightning-fast speed. Instead of going with that flow, change the pace. Chew your food. Make connections. Put the phone away and have a face-to-face conversation instead.

It's what life is and should always be—authentic. Paced. Present.

## THE REALITY

In our society, there are three main problems leading to unhealthy lifestyles:

* Stress

* Toxic food

* Sedentary lifestyle

These are not new phenomena, but they are extremely real and have been shortening lives for decades. Stress has become part of *daily* life. From intense work demands and a taxing home life to money woes and not enough "time in the day," we often put our emphasis on what needs to "get done" rather than spending time with our loved ones and just enjoying it all—even the chaos.

# LIVING THE MEDITERRANEAN LIFESTYLE ANTIDOTE

A little tweaking of your habits and mind-set not only changes your health, it can completely change your life. Here are a few tips for dealing with our modern lifestyles:

## STRESS

**COOK AT LEAST THREE MEALS PER WEEK WITH YOUR FAMILY.** How often do you eat on the run? In your car? At your desk? In front of the television? Alone? Whatever meal it is, put away all distractions and revel in making the meal together. Getting kids and spouses involved is not only a great way to teach how fun cooking can be, but it can be a tradition you begin to look forward to. If you live alone, invite some friends over and cook together. Play some music, share recipes, and enjoy the art of creating a meal to share.

**IF POSSIBLE, TAKE A MIDDAY NAP.** There's a reason companies like Google have nap pods. People are more productive if their bodies can act on 24-hour cycles. Think about babies. They are the epitome of living on a 24-hour clock. They sleep for several hours, are awake for a few, sleep for several hours, are awake for a few, and around and around it goes. Somewhere along the line, we trained ourselves to stay awake all day, every day, for 16 hours at a time. But a short midday nap can repair the body and reset the internal clock so you're more productive in the afternoon.

**MOVE AT A DIFFERENT PACE.** Just because everyone around you is going fast, their heads buried in their phones and computers, doesn't mean you have to. Have you ever watched a child walk down the street or play on the playground? Everything is exciting or new: a bug, a leaf, a stick. They will squeal in delight and pick up random objects. They are present. We are often just concerned with getting from point A to point B in a timely manner. But try this: Don't rush. Be patient. Be mindful. Slow down.

**WORK ON YOUR RELATIONSHIPS.** It's amazing how many of us live with someone we can't seem to "talk" to. We get defensive or distant or just stop giving him/her the benefit of the doubt. Stop worrying and complaining to your friends and talk to your partner about what's bothering you (and vice versa). Have a weekly check-in to see what you can do better, how you succeeded or failed at communicating, and what needs are or are not being met.

**TRY YOGA.** Maybe yoga isn't your thing; maybe you love it. Regardless, we can all take cues from it. The act of deep breathing alone calms the nerves and gets the oxygen flowing, which means less stress for you. If you are more athletic, look for power flow classes. Want to sweat? Try Bikram. There's something for everyone with this practice. Even meditating can work wonders for the psyche.

**ENJOY LIFE.** How can you enjoy life when it's beating you down? Figure out what makes you truly happy and then *do* it. Don't be inspired to try something; don't say "someday." Do something *today* that you enjoy.

**STAY POSITIVE.** Yeah, yeah. We hear it all the time: Think positive! But we are a nation of critical thinkers. We overanalyze, worry, and tend to take a negative approach to certain things. For

---

# GARDENING AND GROWING

You can always find space for a garden, whether it's at a nearby family member's home, on the fire escape, or on the kitchen windowsill. It makes it so gratifying, affordable, and easy to enjoy fresh vegetables and fruit year round. Here are some tips on what to plant in your garden if you're looking to get it started. Vegetables and fruits fall into the categories of warm and cool seasons, depending upon what kind of temperatures they need for growth.

## WARM SEASON CROPS

* Cantaloupe
* Celery
* Cucumber
* Eggplant
* Pumpkin
* Snap Pea
* Sweet Potato
* Tomato
* Watermelon
* Zucchini

## COOL SEASON CROPS

* Arugula
* Asparagus
* Beets
* Broccoli
* Brussels sprouts
* Cabbage
* Carrots
* Cauliflower
* Chard
* Kale
* Lettuce
* Onion
* Spinach

If you don't have a green thumb or lack outdoor space, think about investing in a small herb garden. They are cheap, easy to maintain, and can add a plethora of flavors to your favorite dishes. Growing basil, cilantro, parsley, dill, and oregano is simple and you can do it right in your kitchen.

---

today, try to be positive. Whether you are stuck in traffic or your morning is just going south, have compassion for anyone and everyone you come across, including yourself. When you are faced with a stressful situation, choose the calmer option. Just try it and see how stress disappears from your life.

**SOCIALIZE.** Stop connecting with friends on Facebook, Twitter, or through text messages. Make actual plans and go out. Keep your phones in your bags or leave them at home. Again, be present. Though we are more "connected" than ever, we have also become lonelier and more isolated. Enjoy the people in your life whenever you can.

## TOXIC FOOD

**STOP EATING PROCESSED FOODS.** Go to your pantry or cupboards. See any boxes or packages? What about in the refrigerator—any packaged items in there? Those are probably processed foods. Eating food that comes from the ground or in its most natural state is the way we were meant to eat. Period. Stick to the perimeter of the store and buy foods that have no ingredient list. Can't give up the bread or cereal? Search for items with the least number of ingredients (all of which you can pronounce) and no added sugar or salt. Whenever possible, purchase your nuts, seeds, and grains from bulk bins and not packages or cans.

**BUY ORGANIC.** Why organic? Organic food means that everything from the soil to the produce hasn't been treated with pesticides. Ingested pesticides have proven to be incredibly unhealthy (if they can kill pests, what do you think they can do to you?) and can even compromise the nutrition of a fruit or vegetable. But maybe you can't afford organic food. See "The Dirty Dozen and the Clean Fifteen" (page 20) for tips on which foods are the most important to buy organic, and what you can get away with eating conventionally grown.

**BUY LOCAL.** Another great option is to check out local farmers' markets. When you buy local, you're eating food that's grown closer to home, which means less traveling, storing, and sitting on a shelf, and more nutrition for you. Ask farmers about their practices. Some only spray their produce once or twice per year, or not at all. Many are even organic but can't afford the "certified" organic label.

**EAT FOOD, NOT CALORIES.** Our bodies crave nutrition, not calories. If we fill up on chips, cookies, or candy, our bodies will signal they are still hungry because they need vitamins and minerals. Try and make the bulk of your meals come from actual food from whole sources.

**MAKE HEALTHY SWAPS.** If you have corn oil or canola oil in your house, swap it with extra-virgin olive oil. If you have white rice, swap with quinoa or brown rice. If you have regular pasta, try a whole wheat variety instead (or make your own—see our recipe for Fresh Pasta Dough on page 131). Milk chocolate? Try dark. Canned fruit? Make a smoothie from fresh or frozen fruit. Tons of store-bought condiments? Try fresh herbs or spices instead. Small, effective changes will not only alter your palate, they'll shrink your waistline and boost internal health.

## SEDENTARY LIFESTYLE

**FIND AN ACTIVITY YOU LOVE.** Chances are, there's something you love to do. Maybe you jumped on a trampoline every single day when you were a kid. (Adult gymnastics class.) Maybe you loved the playground. (Obstacle course races.) Maybe you were always in skates or dancing or loved helping your parents with the yard work. Maybe hiking clears your head or maybe you've always been into running. Incorporate the activities you love into your regular routine—whether this is three times a week or seven, every bit counts.

**MAKE EXERCISE A PRIORITY.** Whatever you enjoy doing, make it a priority (even if this means just taking a nice walk after dinner). Find people you admire in sports or activities you love and surround yourself with like-minded individuals who are pursuing the same goals. Make physical activity *just* as important as going to work or paying bills or spending time with your children or socializing. Our bodies will not thrive if we do not move. Period. An active body stays active. A sedentary body will perish.

**SET YOUR TIMER.** If you have a normal desk job, you might feel like all you do is sit, hunched in front of your computer. Set that handy timer on your phone every hour, and get up for a few minutes. Do squats, push-ups, take a walk, go up and down stairs, stretch. Just do something to get the blood flowing. Do this every day.

**FIGURE OUT WHAT MOTIVATES YOU.** Do you enjoy exercising alone? Is it your time to think? Do you want a buddy to train with? Are you competitive? Do you need a group to keep you accountable? Do you want to race for a cause? Figure out what works for you (not against you), and then set the stage so you will be successful. If you know you can't get up and exercise before work, take your lunch hour and hit the gym. If nights are hard, set out your gym clothes, iPod, water, and a preworkout snack the night before so you won't have any excuses not to go when you get up in the morning. Set yourself up for success.

**EVERY TIME YOU HAVE AN OPTION, TAKE THE ACTIVE APPROACH.** If you're ever faced with two options—one sedentary and one active—choose active. Escalator or stairs? Take the stairs. Parking close or far? Park far. Walking to a nearby restaurant or driving? Walk. These small, daily choices can literally change the trajectory of your health.

Remember that health is cumulative. It's not created from one single day or one event. It's the repetitive nature of our unhealthy or healthy habits that will make all the difference for the type of life we lead.

# A FINAL WORD

Whenever you embark on a new way of life or way of eating, remember to take it one component at a time. Perhaps you start with having dinner with your family once a week, or you become more active. Or you make a healthy dietary swap or try one recipe a week from this book. Remember that gradual changes can be more effective and sustainable than trying to change everything at once. This isn't a diet. *Living the Mediterranean Diet* is a way of life.

As you can see, there are innumerable benefits to partaking in *Living the Mediterranean Diet*. To put it simply? You *can* lose weight, erase stress, improve your endurance, and strengthen your confidence (and mood) with the tips and recipes in this book. What are you waiting for? Make smart decisions. Enjoy your food. Enjoy your life.

—Rea Frey

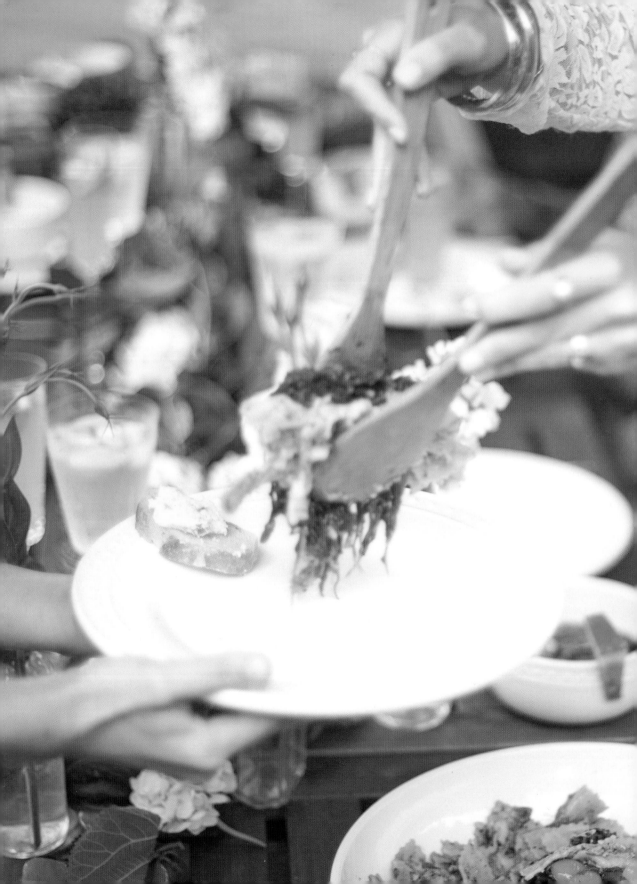

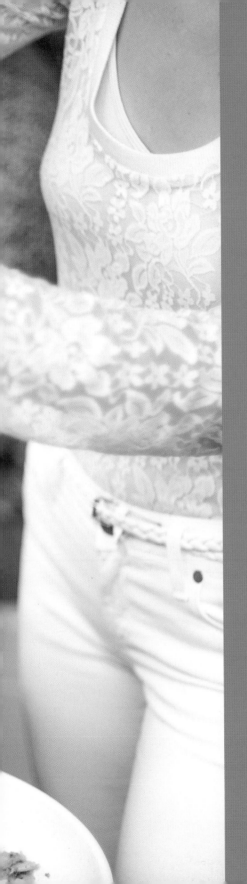

# SPRING

*"Is the spring coming?" he said,*
*"What is it like?"*

*"It is the sun shining on the rain and*
*the rain falling on the sunshine..."*

—Frances Hodgson Burnett,
*The Secret Garden*

The arrival of spring in the Mediterranean (and in our home) is a time for celebration, a time for rebirth and renewal. Paving the way for the seasons to come, spring offers us ever-abounding gifts of freshness: light, leafy greens, fragrant herbs, broccoli, asparagus, sweet peas, and more. For these recipes, we take our very favorite foods and alter them a bit to take full advantage of spring's selection. We give them new twists, like pesto made with sunflower seeds and gazpacho made with watermelon. When the weather is warm, we love to cook with a certain lightness, with less time spent over a hot stove indoors and more time spent in the open air with an outdoor grill. We arrange our flowers, pour our wine, and dine al fresco in a natural and relaxed atmosphere.

# WATERMELON GAZPACHO

GAZPACHO IS A COLD soup made from raw fruits and vegetables that can be smooth or chunky, elegant or casual. It is generally made with tomatoes as the prominent flavor; this recipe, however, honors another beautiful vinelike flowering plant—the watermelon. Gazpacho is a perfect starter for an outdoor lunch or dinner.  SERVES 4 TO 6

- 5 cups roughly chopped watermelon, plus 1 cup chopped, plus 6 small triangles for garnish
- 2 medium hothouse cucumbers, roughly chopped, plus ½ cup finely chopped for garnish
- 1 cup whole baby heirloom tomatoes
- 2 celery stalks, roughly chopped, plus ½ cup finely chopped for garnish
- 7 mint leaves
- 2 tablespoons minced fresh ginger
- 1 jalapeño, seeded
- juice of 1 lime
- a pinch of cayenne pepper
- ½ cup chopped red onion
- 1 tablespoon minced fresh rosemary, plus several sprigs, for garnish
- 2 tablespoons minced fresh parsley
- sea salt
- black pepper

## HOW WE CREATE

Place the 5 cups watermelon, 2 cucumbers, tomatoes, celery, mint, ginger, and jalapeño in a food processor and pulse until smooth.

Pulse in the lime juice, cayenne pepper, and sea salt and black pepper to taste. Transfer the mixture to the refrigerator to chill for a cooler soup. Or, transfer into serving bowls and garnish evenly with chopped watermelon, cucumbers, celery, red onion, rosemary, and parsley. For the final touch, place a short partial sprig of rosemary on top and a watermelon triangle, sliced in the center, to fit over the side of each bowl.

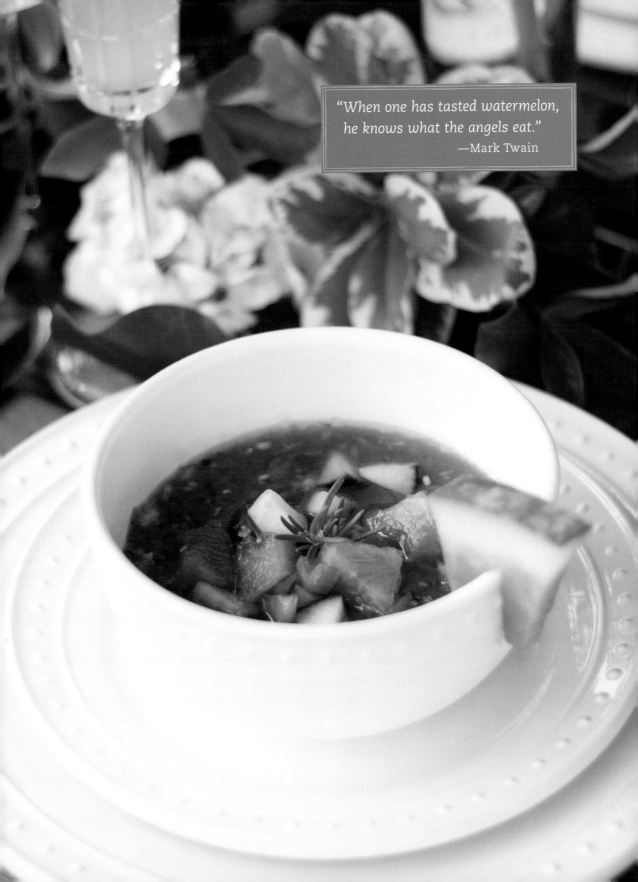

"When one has tasted watermelon,
he knows what the angels eat."
—Mark Twain

# ASPARAGUS, PROSCIUTTO, AND MUSHROOM PIZZA

THERE'S A RESTAURANT we go to in Newport Beach called Canaletto, and they have outrageously tasty pizza. Our favorite pizza is divided into three sections: one for asparagus, one for prosciutto, and one for mushrooms. At first, asparagus seemed like an unlikely pizza topping to us, but after the first bite, we were smitten. If you'd like a healthier pizza, leave the prosciutto out and replace it with something else, like olives, bell peppers, or artichoke hearts. MAKES 2 (10-INCH) PIZZAS (SERVES 4)

## FOR THE SAUCE

2 tablespoons olive oil

2 garlic cloves, minced

2 tablespoons dry red wine

2 tablespoons chopped fresh basil

2 tablespoon minced fresh oregano

1 teaspoon sea salt

½ teaspoon black pepper

1 (28-ounce) can crushed San Marzano tomatoes

## FOR THE PIZZA

1 Fresh Pizza Dough (page 134)

16 ounces (1 pound) whole milk mozzarella, in ½-inch thick slices

2 cups sliced cremini mushrooms

10 asparagus spears, thick bottoms trimmed

6 slices prosciutto (optional)

## HOW WE CREATE

Make the sauce. Warm the olive oil in a medium saucepan over medium-low heat. Add the garlic and red wine, and let simmer. Once they begin to cook, add the basil, oregano, sea salt, and black pepper. Allow to simmer again for about 4 minutes. Add the tomatoes and stir. Let simmer on low for at least 30 minutes, stirring occasionally, until sauce is smooth. If tomato chunks still remain, use a food processor or immersion blender to smooth. Cover with a lid and set aside.

Preheat the oven to 500°F.

Prepare the pizza dough according to the recipe. Top the dough with half the pizza sauce. Arrange half the mozzarella slices, half the mushrooms, half the asparagus spears, and half the prosciutto (if using) however you please. We like to do three sections, like Canaletto does, because it makes us feel like we're having three different pizzas. Bake in the oven for 8 to 10 minutes, until crust is golden.

Repeat for the second pizza.

WELLNESS NOTE: For something different, try eating the asparagus raw while you create your pizza (something we discovered not long ago, but we love it). Asparagus is best and most flavorful in the spring, so for freshness and flavor, make sure to select straight, smooth stalks with tightly closed tips.

# BLACK PEPPERED LAMB CHOPS
## WITH MINT-YOGURT SAUCE

DURING SPECIAL SPRINGTIME OCCASIONS, lamb finds its way to our table as a beautiful and savory centerpiece. In this recipe, the sweet and peppery aroma of mint cuts through the heaviness of the meat and gives the dish a certain lightness in flavor. SERVES 4

### FOR THE SAUCE

1 cup plain whole milk Greek yogurt

juice of 1 lime

grated zest of 1 lemon

2 garlic cloves, chopped

⅓ cup chopped fresh mint leaves

2 tablespoons minced fresh chives

½ teaspoon ground cumin

sea salt

black pepper

### FOR THE LAMB CHOPS

6 lamb chops (about 1½ pounds), ¾-inch thick

6 garlic cloves, chopped

3 tablespoons chopped fresh rosemary

1 teaspoon chopped fresh sage

¼ cup extra-virgin olive oil

1 teaspoon balsamic vinegar

sea salt

black pepper

### HOW WE CREATE

Place all the sauce ingredients in a small bowl and mix well. Add sea salt and black pepper to taste. Refrigerate while you prepare the lamb chops (and up to 2 days).

Rub sea salt and black pepper onto each lamb chop and set aside in a large bowl to marinate at room temperature for 30 minutes to 1 hour. Mix the garlic, rosemary, sage, olive oil, and balsamic vinegar in a small bowl and pour evenly over the lamb chops.

ON THE GRILL: On medium-high heat, grill for about 4 minutes on each side while slowly pouring any leftover marinade on top of the chops. Remove from the heat and allow the meat to cool for 7 minutes before serving with the mint sauce.

IN THE OVEN: Preheat the oven to 400°F. Place the lamb chops in a large ovenproof skillet and sear on medium-high heat for about 3 minutes on each side. Place the skillet with the seared lamb chops in the oven and roast for about 10 minutes. Remove and let cool slightly before serving with the mint sauce.

# FARFALLE PASTA
## WITH ARUGULA, TOMATOES, AND SUNFLOWER SEED PESTO

PESTO IS SO SIMPLE and so versatile. It can be used on pasta, sandwiches, pizza, baked chicken, crostini, and the list goes on. With the price of pine nuts always a little shocking, we developed this recipe with another beloved (and more affordable) option with a similar mild and nutty taste: sunflower seeds. The fresh pasta combines our favorite summer flavors—tomatoes, basil, and arugula. SERVES 4

### FOR THE PESTO

2 cups fresh basil

3 garlic cloves

1 tablespoon raw honey

¼ cup raw shelled sunflower seeds

¾ cup extra-virgin olive oil

1 tablespoon fresh lemon juice (about ½ small lemon)

½ cup grated Pecorino Romano cheese

sea salt

black pepper

### FOR THE PASTA

1 pound Farfalle Fresh Pasta Dough (page 131)

3 cups packed arugula

2 cups halved cherry tomatoes

2 tablespoons extra-virgin olive oil

¼ cup shaved Pecorino Romano cheese

### HOW WE CREATE

To make the pesto, toss the basil, garlic, honey, and sunflower seeds into a food processor and process until blended, then slowly incorporate the olive oil and lemon juice and pulse in the cheese. Season with sea salt and black pepper to taste. Thin the pesto with water, 1 teaspoon at a time, if it is too thick. Use the pesto immediately or place it in a bowl with a drizzle of olive oil on top for storing. Cover and refrigerate for up to 4 days.

Prepare the noodles and cook according to the recipe.

To make the pasta, add the fresh farfalle noodles and pesto to a large pot over low heat. Stir until the noodles are evenly coated. Move the mixture to a large bowl and add arugula, tomatoes and drizzled olive oil on top. Stir to wilt the arugula in the warm pasta, if desired, and garnish with shaved Pecorino Romano.

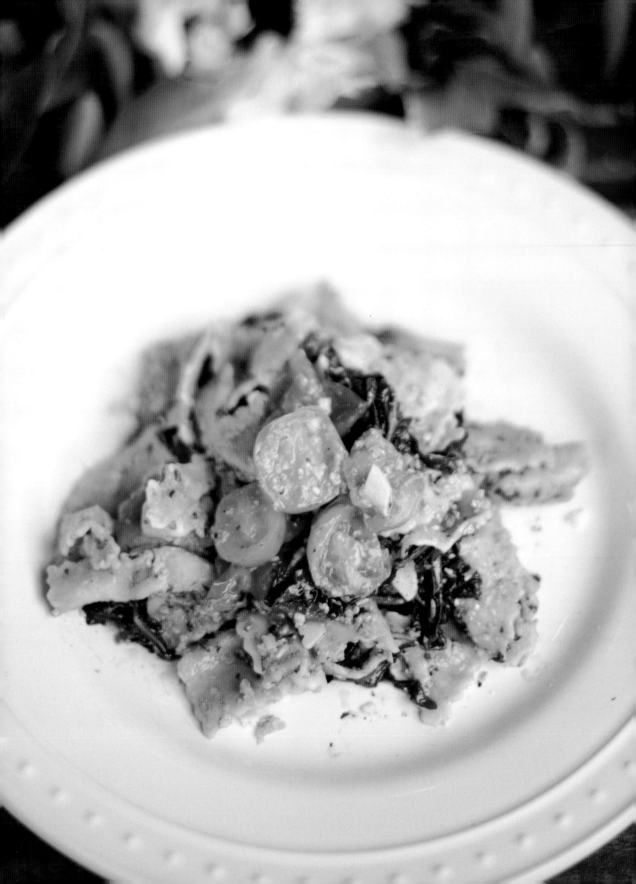

# MEDITERRANEAN CHICKEN STIR-FRY

STIR-FRYING is a wonderfully quick cooking method that seals in the flavors of the foods while also preserving their various colors and textures. It's a popular cooking technique for those evenings when we find our fridge and our energy depleting rapidly. This is a simple dish that combines everything you need in one skillet. It's hearty, clean, and makes great cold leftovers. We make a point to keep chicken and an assortment of vegetables always on hand, so we can whip this up whenever we please. This dish is very versatile and can be served over a bed of brown rice, with sautéed rapini, or mixed with garbanzo beans.  SERVES 4

3 tablespoons extra-virgin olive oil

4 garlic cloves, minced

1 medium sweet yellow onion, roughly chopped

1 tablespoon chopped fresh oregano

2 tablespoons chopped fresh basil

2 tablespoons chopped fresh parsley

1 pound boneless, skinless chicken breasts (3 or 4 breasts), cubed

1 tablespoon white wine vinegar

1 large tomato, chopped

1 cup sliced mushrooms

1 large red bell pepper, chopped

1 large green bell pepper, chopped

2 cups fresh sweet peas

1 teaspoon red pepper flakes

sea salt

black pepper

## HOW WE CREATE

Heat the olive oil in a large skillet over medium heat. Add the garlic, onion, oregano, basil, parsley, and chicken, and cook, stirring, for 4 to 5 minutes, or until the chicken is lightly browned. Add the white wine vinegar and tomato, then the mushrooms, bell peppers, and peas, and sauté for an additional 4 to 5 minutes, stirring frequently. Cover and let simmer on medium-low for about 7 minutes, until vegetables are tender. Add the red pepper flakes and season with sea salt and black pepper to taste.

# BROCCOLI PECAN RAVIOLI

TO GET AWAY from the chaos of daily life, we often visit Nick's mom and stepdad at their tranquil home in the Santa Rosa Mountains of Southern California. One evening, we were preparing for dinner and the trek down the winding mountain roads into town just to go to the grocery store didn't sound too appealing, so we scavenged the fridge, pantry, and garden in an effort to get creative. What we ended up with was this savory ravioli, which now finds itself at the top of the list as one of our favorites. SERVES 4

½ cup extra-virgin olive oil, divided

4 garlic cloves, minced

4 whole green onions, minced

2 carrots, minced

3 celery stalks, minced

¾ cup minced raw pecans, divided

3 cups minced broccoli

2 tablespoons fresh minced rosemary, divided

1 pound Ravioli Fresh Pasta Dough (page 131)

2 tablespoons fresh lemon juice (about 1 small lemon)

¼ cup shaved Parmigiano-Reggiano cheese

sea salt

black pepper

## HOW WE CREATE

Warm ¼ cup of the olive oil in a medium skillet over medium heat. Add the garlic, green onions, carrots, celery, and ½ cup of the pecans. Stir and sauté for about 3 minutes. Add the broccoli, 1 tablespoon rosemary, and sea salt and black pepper to taste. Cook for about 10 minutes, stirring frequently.

Following the ravioli recipe on page 131, use the mixture as filling.

Strain the ravioli into a large serving bowl and mix in the remaining olive oil, lemon juice, pecans, rosemary, and Parmigiano-Reggiano, and season with additional black pepper to taste.

# TUNA STEAKS
## WITH CAPER, OLIVE, AND SUN-DRIED TOMATO RELISH

YOU CAN SUBSTITUTE salmon, swordfish, or halibut for the tuna in this recipe to throw together a simple but sophisticated meal that will soon become a staple in your kitchen (as it did in ours). This can either be made on the grill or roasted in the oven, depending on your preference. The relish can be made a few days ahead of time, if need be, and can also be used as a bruschetta appetizer on top of grilled bread.  SERVES 4

½ cup extra-virgin olive oil, divided

½ cup finely chopped sun-dried tomatoes

¼ cup finely chopped kalamata olives

2 tablespoons fresh lemon juice (about 1 small lemon)

2 tablespoons whole capers, rinsed

2 tablespoons minced fresh parsley

2 teaspoons minced fresh sage

4 (4- to 6-ounce) tuna steaks

sea salt

black pepper

fresh herbs, for garnish

## HOW WE CREATE

In a medium bowl, combine ¼ cup of the olive oil and all of the ingredients except for the tuna, salt, and sage to create the relish. Season with black pepper to taste.

ON THE GRILL: Heat a grill to medium-high. Coat both sides of the tuna with the ¼ cup remaining olive oil and season with sea salt. Grill the tuna steaks on one side until they have good grill marks, about 2 to 4 minutes. Flip the steaks and grill another 2 to 4 minutes, or until the fish flakes when tested with a fork but is still pink in the center. Remove from the heat.

IN THE OVEN: Preheat the oven to 450°F.

Place the tuna steaks on a baking sheet in a single layer. Brush both sides of the tuna with the ¼ cup remaining olive oil and season with sea salt. Bake for 10 to 12 minutes, or until the fish flakes when tested with a fork but is still pink in the center. Remove from oven.

To serve, top the tuna with the relish and garnish with fresh herbs, if you desire. Serve immediately.

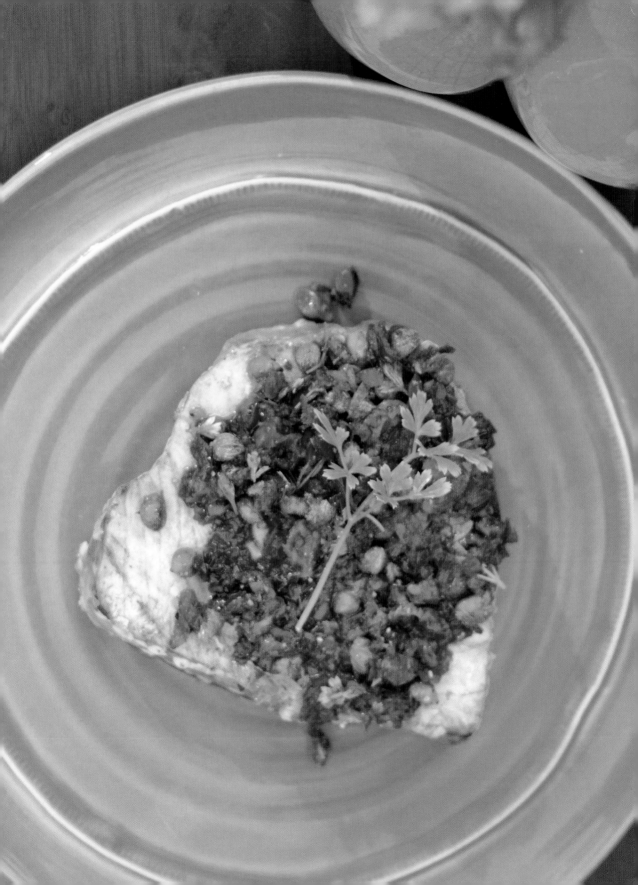

# CAESAR SALAD WITH MESQUITE GRILLED CHICKEN
## AND HOMEMADE DRESSING

IF WE PAY CLOSE ENOUGH ATTENTION to what we are tasting and seeing, the simple and subtle colors and flavors of a fresh, completely homemade Caesar salad can be extraordinary. Here, we use Greek yogurt to replace the egg yolks in the dressing and whole wheat bread for the croutons. It's divine.  SERVES 4

### FOR THE CHICKEN

1 pound boneless, skinless chicken breasts (3 or 4 breasts)

2 tablespoons lemon juice (about 1 small lemon)

3 tablespoons extra-virgin olive oil

2 tablespoons raw honey

1 tablespoon minced fresh parsley

¼ teaspoon cayenne pepper

sea salt

black pepper

### FOR THE DRESSING

⅓ cup plain whole milk Greek yogurt

2 anchovy fillets, mashed

1 garlic clove, minced

2 tablespoons fresh lemon juice (about 1 small lemon)

2 teaspoons whole-grain Dijon mustard

2 tablespoons extra-virgin olive oil

2 tablespoons freshly grated Parmigiano-Reggiano cheese

1 tablespoon chopped fresh chives

sea salt

black pepper

### FOR THE CROUTONS

2 cups torn whole wheat bread

3 tablespoons extra-virgin olive oil

sea salt

black pepper

### FOR THE SALAD

2 heads romaine lettuce, outer leaves removed

Parmigiano-Reggiano cheese, for garnish

## HOW WE CREATE

Marinate the chicken by combining all the ingredients, including the chicken, in a large bowl. Cover the bowl and let sit in refrigerator for at least 20 minutes.

Make the dressing. In a small bowl, whisk together all of the ingredients. Place in the refrigerator until ready to serve the salad.

To make the croutons, preheat the oven to 375°F.

Toss the bread with the olive oil on a baking sheet and season with sea salt and black pepper. Bake, tossing occasionally, for 10 to 15 minutes, or until golden. Let cool.

Meanwhile, remove the chicken from the refrigerator and grill over 100 percent lump mesquite charcoal over medium heat for about 7 minutes per side, or until the chicken is cooked through.

In a large bowl, place the croutons on top of the whole romaine leaves, gently toss with enough dressing to cover the lettuce. Divide the mixture evenly among four plates.

Cut the chicken breasts into strips to place on top of each plate. Garnish each serving with thinly shaved pieces of Parmigiano-Reggiano.

# ROASTED VEGGIE TOWER

HOW CAN IT BE that the simple act of stacking vibrantly colored roasted vegetables on a skewer can rapidly transform even the most timid of cooks into the most gourmet of chefs? We drizzle our veggie towers with marinara sauce (see recipe on page 85) and a sprinkle of Parmigiano-Reggiano. SERVES 4

4 medium portobello mushrooms, stems removed

1 medium eggplant, thickly sliced

2 medium red bell peppers, thickly sliced

1 small red onion, sliced into thick rounds

2 medium zucchini, thickly sliced

¼ cup extra-virgin olive oil

¼ cup dry white wine

2 garlic cloves, minced

1 tablespoon lemon juice (about ½ small lemon)

1 tablespoon minced fresh rosemary, plus more for garnish

1 tablespoon minced fresh parsley, plus more for garnish

sea salt

black pepper

## HOW WE CREATE

In a large bowl, combine all of the ingredients. Cover and let marinate for 30 minutes in the refrigerator.

While the veggies are marinating, place four 8-inch skewers in warm water and soak for 20 minutes.

Preheat the oven to 425°F.

Remove the veggies from the refrigerator and stack the ingredients on the wooden skewers in the following order: mushroom, eggplant, red pepper, red onion, eggplant, and zucchini.

Bake for 20 minutes and garnish with more rosemary and parsley, if desired.

WELLNESS NOTE: Did you know that you can eat zucchini blossoms? Zucchini grows from a golden blossom that blooms underneath the leaves. These blooms (like the blooms of pumpkins) can be eaten in a variety of ways, including stuffed and in salads. You may not be able to find zucchini blossoms at the grocery store, so try a stroll to your local farmers' market during late spring and throughout the summer. Or grow them yourself—it's an easy addition to your garden that will have you making all things zucchini.

# BALSAMIC-MARINATED PORTOBELLO MUSHROOMS

PORTOBELLO MUSHROOMS are simply cremini mushrooms that have been allowed to mature, with a dense, meaty texture and intense earthy flavor. Look for portobello mushrooms that are plump, firm, and brown in color, and stray from mushrooms that are slimy, wrinkled, or have spots. These are a great meat replacement on a whole wheat bun and pair well with an evening salad (like Caesar Salad with Mesquite Grilled Chicken and Homemade Dressing on page 42, as the flavors combine to form a uniquely hearty meal). SERVES 4

4 large portobello mushrooms, stems removed

4 garlic cloves, minced

3 tablespoons chopped fresh chives

⅓ cup balsamic vinegar

¼ cup extra-virgin olive oil

sea salt

black pepper

## HOW WE CREATE

Clean the mushrooms with a damp cloth. Mix all of the ingredients together in a large bowl and marinate mushrooms for at least 25 minutes.

ON THE GRILL: Preheat the grill to medium-high heat. Place the marinated mushrooms on the grill top-side down. Drizzle half of the remaining marinade over mushrooms and grill for about 4 minutes on one side, or until grill marks are visible. Repeat on the other side.

IN THE OVEN: Preheat the oven to 400°F. Place the marinated mushrooms top-side down in an ovensafe baking dish. Pour the remaining marinade over the mushrooms and roast for 10 minutes. Turn and roast until the mushrooms are browned and tender, about 15 minutes.

# MEDITERRANEAN RICE SALAD

THIS IS A REFRESHING SALAD with incredible flavors. We use any leftovers we may have and serve them alongside grilled chicken for lunch the following day.  SERVES 4

½ cup extra-virgin olive oil, divided

1 cup long-grain brown rice

2 cups water

¼ cup fresh lemon juice (about 2 small lemons)

1 garlic clove, minced

1 teaspoon minced fresh rosemary

1 teaspoon minced fresh mint

3 Belgian endives, chopped

1 medium red bell pepper, chopped

1 medium hothouse cucumber, chopped

½ cup chopped whole green onion

½ cup chopped kalamata olives

¼ teaspoon red pepper flakes

¾ cup crumbled feta cheese

sea salt

black pepper

## HOW WE CREATE

In a medium saucepan over low heat, add ¼ cup of the olive oil, the rice, and a pinch of sea salt, and stir to coat the rice. Add the water and let simmer until the water is absorbed, stirring occasionally. Pour the rice into a large bowl to let it cool.

In a separate large bowl, mix together the lemon juice, garlic, rosemary, mint, endives, bell pepper, cucumber, green onion, olives, red pepper flakes, and the remaining ¼ cup olive oil. Add the rice to the mixture and toss to combine. Gently mix in the feta cheese. Taste and add sea salt and black pepper, if needed.

# SWISS CHARD CHARDONNAY SAUTÉ

WE PLANTED SWISS CHARD in our garden from seed and, like proud parents, we have loved watching it unfold and grow into an array of colors and sizes. We call it the filet mignon of the leafy greens, as it literally melts in your mouth. SERVES 4

1 large bunch Swiss chard

¼ cup extra-virgin olive oil

1 medium sweet yellow onion, roughly chopped

5 garlic cloves, sliced

¼ cup chardonnay

sea salt

black pepper

## HOW WE CREATE

Trim 1 to 2 inches off the stems of the chard and discard. Warm the olive oil in a large skillet over medium heat, add the onion and garlic,and let cook for 3 minutes. Add the chard, chardonnay, and a touch of sea salt and black pepper. Cover the skillet with a lid and let cook for about 3 minutes. Remove the lid and stir frequently until the chard stems are tender, about 7 more minutes.

# LEMON-THYME SORBET
# IN LEMON CUPS

WITH A FRESH HINT of thyme, this very-lemon sorbet will spring you into the season of citrus and blossoms and shed any shade of winter blues you may have acquired in the previous months. SERVES 4

- 1 cup raw honey, plus 1 tablespoon for drizzling on top (optional)
- 1 cup water

- 1½ cups freshly squeezed lemon juice (from about 12 small lemons, with 4 lemon halves reserved to use as cups)
- 1 large bunch fresh thyme, tied with a kitchen string, plus a few sprigs for garnish

## HOW WE CREATE

Combine the honey, water, and lemon juice in a large saucepan over medium heat and stir until the honey is dissolved. Remove from the heat, add the thyme, and allow the flavors to infuse for about 3 hours in the saucepan with the lid on.

Pour the lemon mixture into your ice cream maker and freeze according to the manufacturer's instructions.

While the sorbet is churning, cut a small circular slice off the bottoms of the reserved lemon halves so as to make them stand up, then use a small spoon to hollow out the insides. Transfer the sorbet into the lemon cups. Garnish each with a sprig of thyme and a drizzle of honey, if desired. Serve immediately or store in the freezer for later enjoyment.

> WELLNESS NOTE: Lemons are rich in Vitamin C. We squeeze fresh lemon into our water, onto our salads, and into our sorbet whenever the opportunity presents itself.

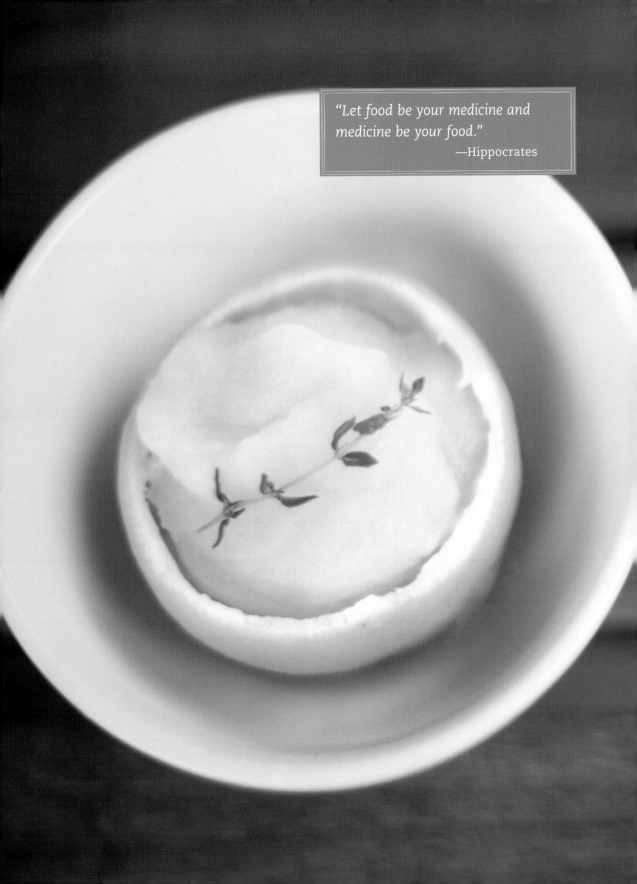

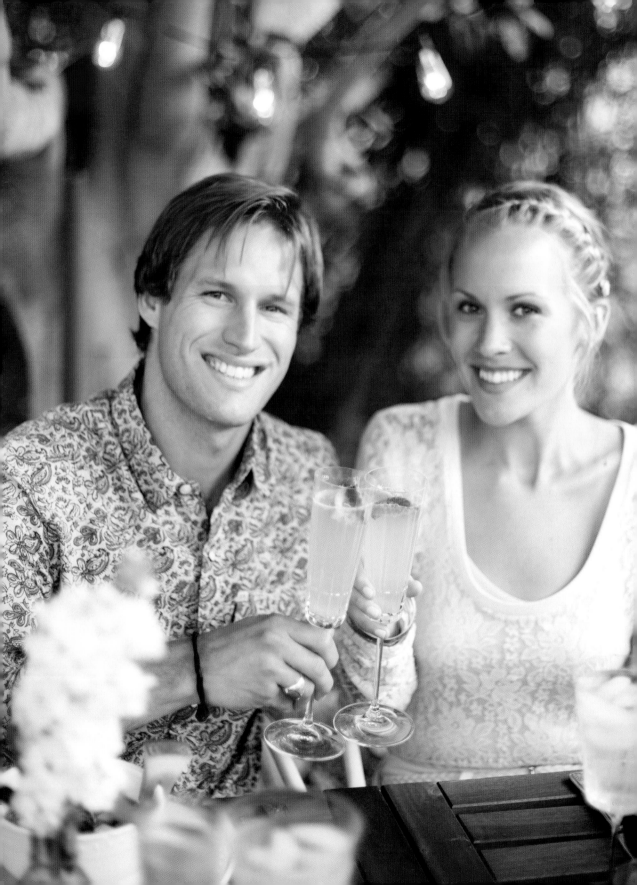

# GRAPEFRUIT MINT PROSECCO

PROSECCO IS AN ITALIAN sparking white wine that is generally dry or extra-dry. We find it to be a tastier and less expensive alternative to champagne (especially when combined with fresh grapefruit juice and grapefruit mint from our garden). If you're new to proscecco, try the Cupcake brand, found in most markets for about $10 a bottle. A slightly pricier bottle of La Marca, which in and of itself has the tantalizing grapefruit-filled tones of spring, is our go-to splurge. We recommend serving this drink with a late afternoon meal outdoors in the sunshine. Cheers! SERVES 6

- 1 (750-milliliter) bottle prosecco, chilled
- ¾ cup fresh grapefruit juice (about 1 large grapefruit)
- 12 fresh grapefruit mint leaves (or any variety of fresh mint)

## HOW WE CREATE

Fill champagne flutes three-quarters full with prosecco and top with fresh grapefruit juice. Garnish each flute with 2 mint leaves.

> WELLNESS NOTE: Although it's often tempting to go for the ease of store-bought grapefruit juice, we strongly encourage squeezing your own. Fresh-squeezed grapefruit juice is good for the metabolism and is full of vitamin C, vitamin A, and potassium. Plus, it tastes wonderful when paired with bubbles.

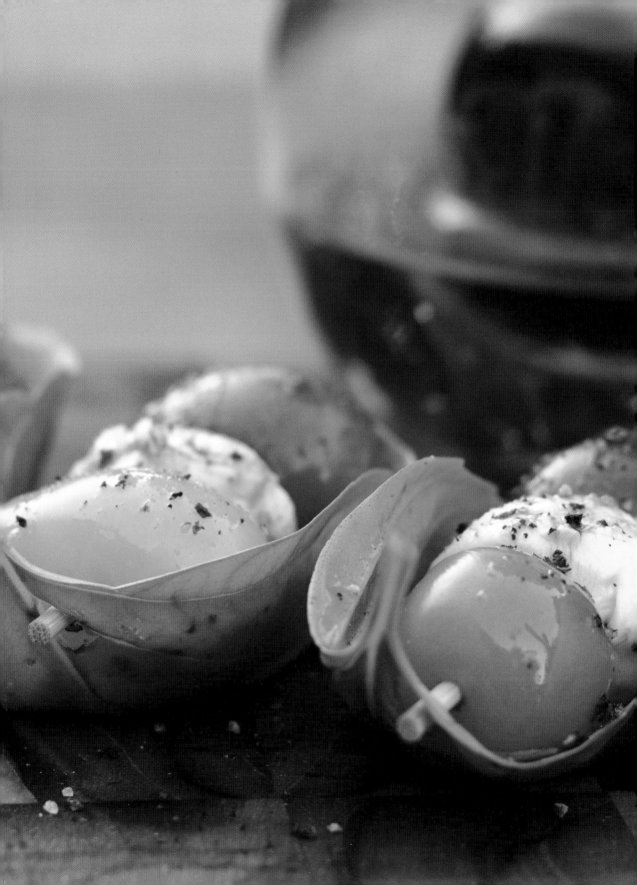

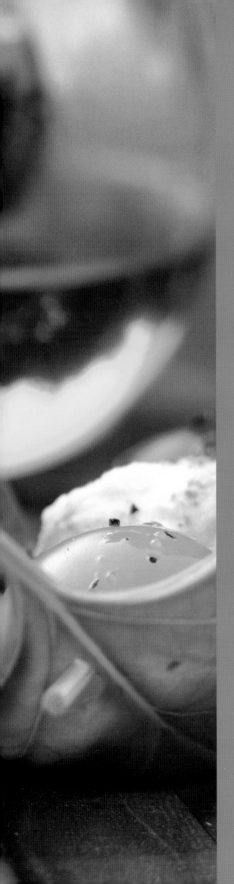

# SUMMER

*"And so with the sunshine and the great bursts of leaves growing on the trees, just as things grow in fast movies, I had that familiar conviction that life was beginning over again with the summer."*

—F. Scott Fitzgerald, *The Great Gatsby*

Summer is a time for eating fruit fresh off the trees in the backyard, for cleansing ourselves in the salt of the sea and the ocean breeze, for fresh and natural flavors to be enjoyed in the sunshine followed by the occasional treat. Summer means growth and goodness, a time when tomatoes and melon are eaten daily and fresh fish flourish. Cucumbers, figs, kale, and eggplant make their way into our recipes and we enjoy eating outside in the late evening as the sun is setting, surrounded by good people, good red wine, and good tunes.

# CAPRESE BOATS

NOTHING SAYS SUMMERTIME like caprese. We love the simplicity of grabbing handfuls of basil from the garden and pairing them with the first of the season's ripe tomatoes.  MAKES 8 BOATS (SERVES 4)

8 large fresh basil leaves

16 cherry tomatoes, red, orange, and yellow mix

8 small mozzarella balls

¼ cup extra-virgin olive oil

¼ cup balsamic vinegar

sea salt

black pepper

## HOW WE CREATE

Using 8 mini wooden skewers, pierce one end of each of the basil leaves and push back, allowing room to fit a tomato, followed by a mozzarella ball, and another tomato to create your boat. Then pierce the other end of the basil leaf through the skewer so that the tomatoes and mozzarella are being cradled by the leaf. Drizzle evenly with olive oil and balsamic vinegar, and season with sea salt and black pepper to taste.

> "Everything carries me to you, as if everything that exists, aromas, light, metals, were little boats that sail toward those isles of yours that wait for me."
>
> —Pablo Neruda

# CHILLED AVOCADO-CUCUMBER SOUP

WE LOVE CUCUMBER SOUP so much. What we love especially about this one is the importance the final touches play in the taste and the appearance: the half of an avocado, the sprinkle of turmeric, and the pinch of cayenne pepper add something special to this dish. Although it's light and refreshing, it's filling as well—perfect for a summer lunch. If you prefer less avocado, feel free to reduce the amount to 1 rather than 2 whole avocados.  SERVES 4

2 medium hothouse cucumbers, halved, seeded, and chopped

1½ cups plain whole milk Greek yogurt

2 small shallots, chopped

1 garlic clove, chopped

¼ cup loosely packed chopped fresh parsley

2 tablespoons chopped chives

⅓ cup loosely packed fresh dill sprigs, plus 1 tablespoon for garnish

4 fresh mint leaves, chopped

2 tablespoons fresh lemon juice (about 1 small lemon)

1 tablespoon white wine vinegar

FOR THE GARNISH

2 avocados, halved

4 pinches ground turmeric

4 pinches cayenne pepper

sea salt

black pepper

## HOW WE CREATE

Combine all the soup ingredients in a blender. Blend until smooth. Cover and refrigerate for at least 4 hours. Divide into four bowls.

Top each bowl with half an avocado, a pinch each of turmeric and cayenne pepper, and sea salt and black pepper, to taste.

# CUCUMBER SALAD WITH CRUMBLED FETA AND PINE NUTS

THIS TRADITIONAL SUMMER SALAD is great for a quick and healthy lunch. Feel free to substitute black beans for the garbanzo beans and sunflower seeds for the pine nuts.  SERVES 4

2 medium hothouse cucumbers, cubed

3 whole green onions, chopped

1 (15-ounce) can garbanzo beans, or 1½ cups home-cooked garbanzo beans

½ cup crumbled feta cheese

½ cup pine nuts

3 tablespoons fresh lemon juice (about 1½ small lemons)

2 tablespoons chopped fresh parsley

¼ cup extra-virgin olive oil

sea salt

black pepper

## HOW WE CREATE

Gently mix all the ingredients together in a large bowl, seasoning with sea salt and black pepper to taste. Divide the salad among four small bowls (or mason jars). Feel free to garnish with extra olive oil and add more sea salt and black pepper to taste, if desired.

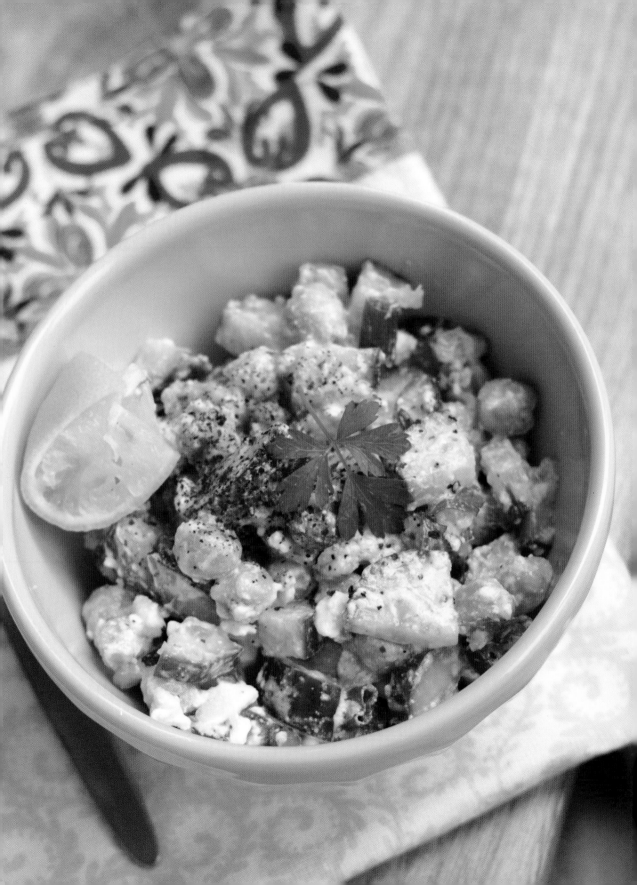

# GRILLED PROSCIUTTO E MELONE

PROSCIUTTO MEANS SO MUCH more to us than simply a paper-thin salted and cured ham. It's an Italian classic, delicate in texture and rich in taste, a treat that sometimes finds its way into our kitchen on special occasions or a seemingly idle summer afternoon. To cut down on the saturated fat, feel free to use half the amount of prosciutto by dividing each slice in half.  SERVES 4

½ medium cantaloupe, sliced into 8 wedges

½ medium honeydew melon, sliced into 8 wedges

16 large basil leaves (1 per melon slice)

16 slices prosciutto (1 per melon slice)

2 tablespoons extra-virgin olive oil

black pepper

Balsamic Reduction (optional, page 93)

## HOW WE CREATE

Heat a grill to medium-high. Place 1 basil leaf on each piece of melon and wrap with 1 piece of prosciutto. Skewers are not necessary, although you can stick them through the melon if you feel so inclined. Drizzle each slice with olive oil (making sure to coat both sides), and top them with a sprinkle of black pepper. Throw them on the barbecue and sear until you see grill marks, 3 to 4 minutes per side. Add more black pepper as well as a drizzle of the Balsamic Reduction, if desired.

If you don't have a grill, serve the wrapped melons raw or cook them in a skillet on high heat and sear until golden.

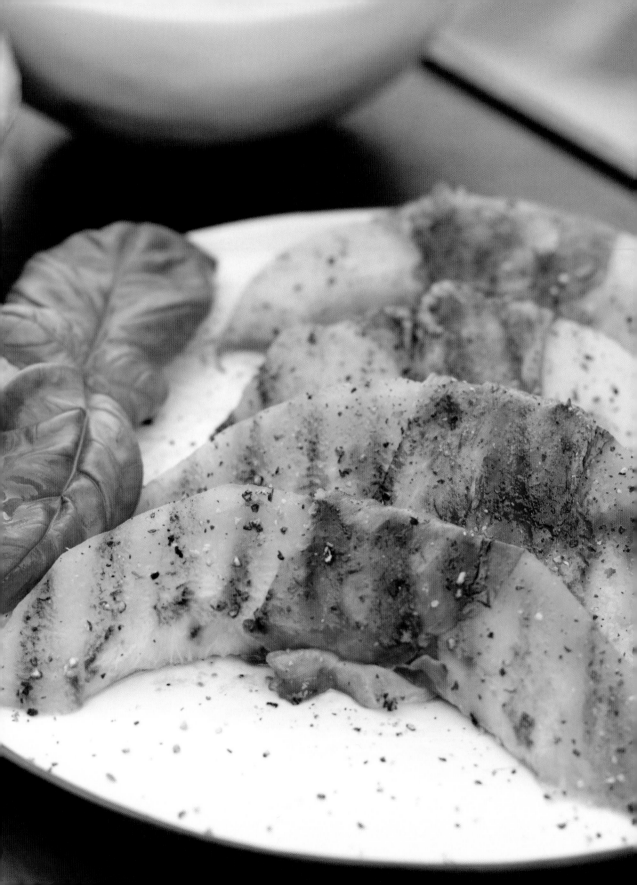

# AVOCADO AND LIME SHRIMP COCKTAIL

GROWING UP on an avocado farm, it seemed to be a house rule that we try every food item with an avocado to accompany it, at least once. One of the first times Nick came to the farm, I insisted that my mom make her avocado and secret sauce shrimp cocktail. She did and, as I expected, Nick loved it. We change the recipe around a bit when we make it ourselves, using fresh tomatoes in place of ketchup and Greek yogurt instead of mayo to give the sauce a fresh and healthy spin. And of course, for my mother's approval, we never fail to add the avo. —*Bay* SERVES 4

## FOR THE SHRIMP

- 16 fresh jumbo shrimp, peeled and deveined
- 2 tablespoons fresh lime juice (about 1 large lime)
- 1 garlic clove, minced
- ¼ teaspoon cayenne pepper
- sea salt
- black pepper

## FOR THE SAUCE

- 1 tablespoon fresh lime juice (about ½ large lime)
- 2 cups cherry tomatoes
- ½ cup plain whole milk Greek yogurt
- 1 tablespoon whole-grain mustard
- 1 teaspoon raw honey
- 3 tablespoons chopped fresh parsley
- sea salt
- black pepper

## FOR THE GARNISH

- 2 large avocados (preferably Hass), cut into small cubes
- 4 lime wedges
- 2 tablespoons chopped fresh parsley
- black pepper

## HOW WE CREATE

Soak four 8-inch wooden skewers in warm water for 20 minutes.

To prepare the shrimp, in a medium bowl, combine the shrimp, lime juice, garlic, and cayenne pepper. Cover the bowl, allowing the mixture to marinate in the refrigerator for 30 to 45 minutes, stirring occasionally.

While the shrimp is marinating, prepare the sauce. Put all ingredients in a food processor and blend until smooth. Set aside.

Remove the shrimp from the marinade and thread onto the skewers (there should be 4 shrimp per skewer). Sprinkle with sea salt and black pepper.

ON THE GRILL: Heat a grill to medium-high heat. Grill the shrimp skewers on one side until you see grill marks, 1 to 3 minutes depending on the heat of your barbecue. Flip the skewers over to repeat on the other side, and pour the remainder of the marinade onto the shrimp. Grill for 1 to 3 more minutes on the second side.

IN THE OVEN: Preheat the oven to 400°F.

Place the skewers on a baking sheet and bake for 4 to 6 minutes, turning them once, until the shrimp are pink and tender.

To serve, divide the cocktail sauce evenly among four wine or martini glasses and place 4 shrimp in each glass. Garnish with avocado, lime wedges, fresh parsley, and a sprinkle of black pepper.

WELLNESS NOTE: Also known as the "alligator pear," the avocado is high in heart-healthy monounsaturated fat and is a surprisingly great replacement for butter or oil in baked goods. Avocados are known to make your skin glow and hair shine. We try to eat one every day of the season—it's a great snack-on-the-go with a sprinkle of sea salt and black pepper.

# WILD SALMON ON PECAN WOOD WITH DILL-YOGURT SAUCE

SUMMER MEANS SALMON. We recommend you buy fresh, wild salmon. It might be a little pricier, but it's worth the splurge—it's a healthier and tastier choice than frozen or farm-raised salmon. So light up the grill, enjoy the outdoors, and take advantage of what nature has to offer you. SERVES 4

## FOR THE SAUCE

¾ cup plain whole milk Greek yogurt

3 teaspoons whole-grain Dijon mustard

2 tablespoons fresh lemon juice (about 1 small lemon)

1 tablespoon minced fresh dill

1 tablespoon whole capers, rinsed

sea salt

black pepper

## FOR THE SALMON

¼ cup extra-virgin olive oil

2 tablespoons fresh lemon juice (about 1 small lemon)

4 (4- to 6-ounce) salmon fillets

4 tablespoons minced fresh dill, plus extra sprigs for garnish

sea salt

black pepper

## HOW WE CREATE

Prepare the sauce by combining all the ingredients and set aside.

ON THE GRILL: Prepare your barbecue with natural charcoal and pecan wood. Once the grill has reached medium-low heat, prepare the salmon by brushing olive oil on both sides and squeezing lemon juice on top. Place the fillets skin-side down on the grill and top with the minced dill, and sea salt and black pepper to taste. Cook with lid closed until the edge of the salmon flakes with a fork, about 9 minutes, depending on the thickness of the salmon. Garnish with dill sprigs. Serve immediately along with the sauce.

IN THE OVEN: Preheat your oven to 450°F. Prepare the salmon by brushing olive oil on both sides and squeezing lemon juice on top. Place the fillets skin-side down in a large oven-proof dish and top with the minced dill, and sea salt and black pepper to taste. Bake for 15 minutes, or until the fish flakes with a fork. Garnish with dill sprigs. Serve immediately along with the sauce.

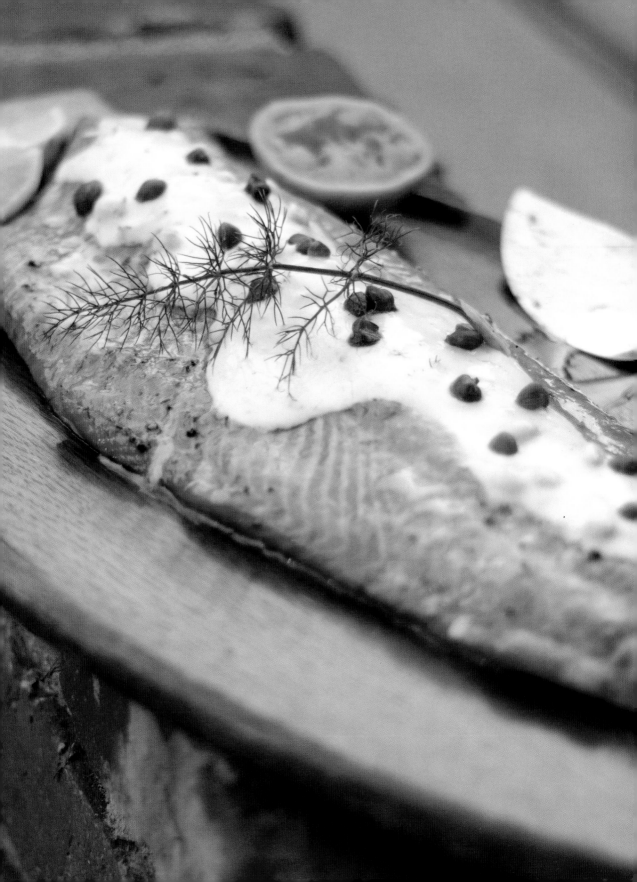

# ORANGE AND FENNEL SALAD WITH WHITE WINE CITRUS DRESSING

WE EAT FENNEL YEAR ROUND, whether it's by itself or included in soups, salads, and pastas—we just love it. This salad brings together the clean flavors of orange, basil, white wine, and lemon juice, a perfect combination for a warm day. Throw it in your picnic basket or serve it on your outdoor table with a glass of iced tea. SERVES 4

## FOR THE DRESSING

2 tablespoons dry white wine

2 tablespoons fresh lemon juice (about 1 small lemon)

¼ cup extra-virgin olive oil

sea salt

black pepper

## FOR THE SALAD

3 oranges, peeled and sliced in rounds

1 large fennel bulb, thinly sliced

½ small red onion, sliced in rounds

12 large fresh basil leaves

## HOW WE CREATE

Whisk the dressing ingredients together in a small bowl, seasoning with sea salt and pepper to taste.

On a large platter, lay the orange slices down and top with fennel, red onion, and fresh basil leaves. Drizzle the dressing over the salad and garnish with a little extra black pepper.

WELLNESS NOTE: Fennel has been used for culinary and medicinal purposes in the Mediterranean for centuries. It helps relieve indigestion, strengthen the immune system, and is often a component of mouth fresheners and toothpastes. It's very rich in potassium and vitamin C. We tend to eat a piece of raw fennel before bed as a calming way to cleanse at the end of the day.

# ALMOND BAKED HALIBUT WITH TOMATO-CAPER SAUCE

TO US, HALIBUT IS LIKE A FINE WINE—something we splurge on only occasionally, and when we do, we make an event out of it. We plan our meal, venture to the local seafood market, and get lost in the buttery goodness of a favorite fish and a favorite dish. SERVES 4

## FOR THE HALIBUT

⅓ cup extra-virgin olive oil

1 tablespoon fresh lemon juice (about ½ small lemon)

¼ cup crushed raw almonds

1 teaspoon raw honey

3 tablespoons minced fresh thyme

4 (4- to 6-ounce) halibut fillets

sea salt

black pepper

## FOR THE SAUCE

¼ cup extra-virgin olive oil

2 garlic cloves, minced

2 cups finely chopped baby heirloom tomatoes

2 tablespoons whole capers, rinsed

½ teaspoon sea salt, plus more to taste

½ teaspoon black pepper, plus more to taste

## HOW WE CREATE

Preheat oven to 400°F.

Toss together the olive oil, lemon juice, almonds, honey, and thyme in a small bowl. Place halibut in a large baking pan lightly coated with olive oil. Season each piece of halibut with a touch of sea salt and black pepper, then evenly spread the almond mixture over the 4 pieces of fish. Bake until fish is cooked through and flakes easily, about 15 minutes.

While the halibut is baking, prepare the side sauce. In a medium skillet, warm the olive oil over medium heat and sauté the garlic for 2 minutes, until fragrant. Add the tomatoes, capers, and at least ½ teaspoon each of sea salt and pepper. Stir occasionally until the tomatoes become soft, about 10 minutes. Remove from the heat.

Remove the halibut from the oven, carefully lift out the fillets, and serve immediately along with the side sauce.

# EGGPLANT AND KALAMATA ROLLS

TENDER AND RICH, these delicate rolled appetizers fill every taste bud with a mouthful of Mediterranean flavor. Though they're small, they're not to be underestimated, as these rolls are filling and bold both in presentation and taste. SERVES 4

1 cup crumbled feta cheese

¼ cup pitted and chopped kalamata olives

2 tablespoons chopped fresh parsley

2 tablespoons chopped fresh chives

2 tablespoons chopped fresh basil

½ teaspoon red pepper flakes

2 large eggplants, sliced lengthwise, ½ inch thick

½ cup extra-virgin olive oil

sea salt

black pepper

## HOW WE CREATE

In a small bowl, combine the feta, kalamata olives, parsley, chives, basil, and red pepper flakes, and set aside.

Brush both sides of the eggplant slices lightly with olive oil.

ON THE GRILL: Heat the grill to medium-high heat. Season the eggplant with salt and pepper. Grill on one side until you see grill marks, about 3 minutes, then flip the slices and grill until tender, about 2 minutes more. Remove from the grill.

IN THE OVEN: Preheat the oven to 450°F. Bake until golden brown on one side, about 7 minutes, then flip the slices over and bake for another 7 minutes, or until golden brown on the second side. Remove from the oven.

ASSEMBLING THE ROLLS: When the eggplant is cool enough to handle, spoon approximately 1 tablespoon of the olive mixture onto the wider end of each slice. Carefully and tightly roll the eggplant slice around the filling, securing the piece in the center with a toothpick. Serve immediately.

# MEDITERRANEAN CEVICHE

CEVICHE IS A SIMPLE DISH made with raw seafood that's cut into small pieces and cooked in the acidity of lime or lemon juice for a few hours. The key to making good ceviche (no matter what ingredients you may choose) is to buy good, fresh fish. Some of our favorite choices are wild-caught cod, tuna, snapper, swordfish, scallops, and shrimp. Ceviche can be eaten as a snack, appetizer, or a meal on its own, served with pita chips, toasted pita bread, or by itself.  SERVES 4

- 1 pound finely diced fresh fish and/or shellfish
- 1 cup fresh lime or lemon juice (about 8 small lemons or 8 large limes)
- 2 cloves garlic, minced
- 1 small red onion, chopped
- 2 large tomatoes, chopped

- 1 small avocado, cut into cubes
- 2 tablespoons minced fresh parsley, plus 1 teaspoon for garnish
- 2 tablespoons minced fresh basil, plus 1 whole leaf for garnish
- sea salt
- black pepper

## HOW WE CREATE

In a large glass bowl, combine the seafood, lemon or lime juice, and garlic, and toss gently to combine. Cover and refrigerate for at least 45 minutes, until the fish no longer looks raw and is "cooked" to your liking. Remove from the refrigerator and drain the liquid through a colander. Transfer the fish back into the bowl and fold in the onion, tomatoes, avocado, parsley, and basil until fully incorporated. Season with sea salt and black pepper to taste. Garnish with extra parsley and basil, and serve immediately.

> WELLNESS NOTE: In ceviche, the acidic juice chemically changes the proteins in the same way heat would. You can marinate your fish in any citrus juice—tangerine, grapefruit, and orange juices are fun to experiment with too.

# HEIRLOOM TOMATO AND KALE PIZZA WITH HERB PIZZA DOUGH

IN THE SUMMERTIME, there's nothing like venturing to the garden or the farmers' market to pick a few heirloom tomatoes, some fresh kale, and an assortment of herbs to create this pizza. Once baked, it turns into a crusted kale-chip glory. We are continuously surprised by just how unique this simple pizza tastes.  MAKES 2 (10-INCH) PIZZAS (SERVES 4)

Fresh Pizza Dough (page 134)

1 tablespoon minced fresh rosemary

1 tablespoon minced fresh basil

1 tablespoon minced fresh parsley

¼ cup extra-virgin olive oil, plus 1 tablespoon for the baking sheet

1 large heirloom tomato, thinly sliced

2 tablespoons chopped fresh thyme

2 cups chopped kale

¼ cup grated Parmigiano-Reggiano cheese

sea salt

black pepper

## HOW WE CREATE

Prepare the pizza dough according to the directions, mixing 1 tablespoon each of minced fresh rosemary, basil, and parsley into the dough before kneading it.

Preheat the oven to 500°F.

Lightly coat the baking sheet with olive oil. Roll the pizza dough out onto the sheet and spread 1 tablespoon olive oil evenly over each pizza. Place half the sliced heirloom tomatoes on top of each pizza followed by half the thyme and kale. Drizzle 1 more tablespoon olive oil over the kale on each pizza, along with half the cheese, salt, and pepper.

Bake for 8 to 10 minutes, or until the crust is golden brown.

Serve immediately.

> WELLNESS NOTE: No need to fear the bold colors and diverse shapes of the quirky heirloom tomato when purchasing or growing them. Accept that they are supposed to have bumps and lines and wildly different physical appearances (just like we do)!

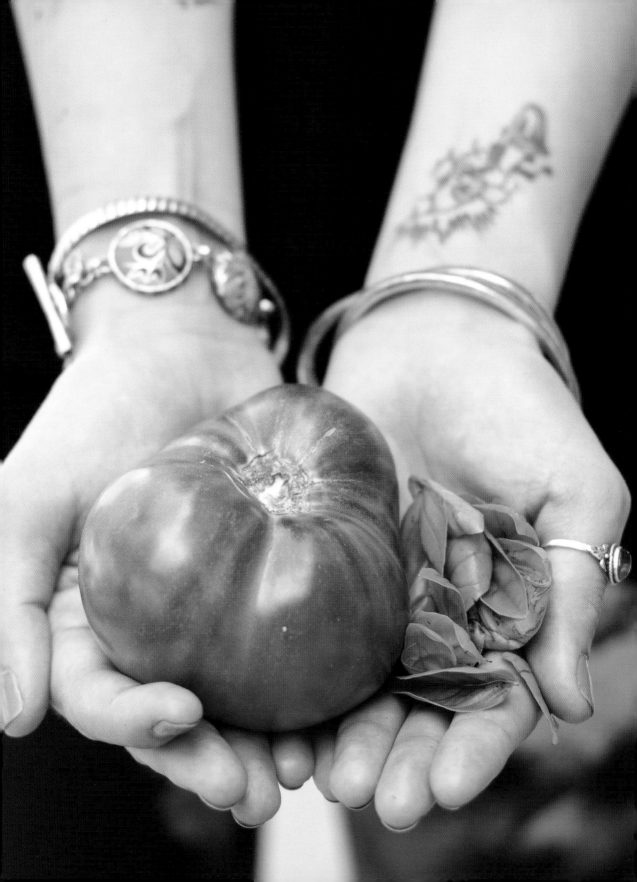

# GARLIC-HERB RICE

USUALLY WHEN WE THINK of rice, it's simple and bland. It's supposed to be that way, right? We used to think this too, until we were inspired by our good pal Gerardo Sanchez, an expert in Peruvian cuisine, partying with pisco, and concocting anything from apple pie to cow hearts in the brick smoker he built by hand. Once we were introduced to Gerry's way of making rice, we could never make *just rice* ever again. SERVES 4

½ cup extra-virgin olive oil, divided

5 large garlic cloves, minced

2 cups brown jasmine rice

4 cups water

1 teaspoon sea salt

1 teaspoon black pepper

3 tablespoons chopped fresh chives

2 tablespoons chopped fresh parsley

1 tablespoon chopped fresh basil

## HOW WE CREATE

Add ¼ cup of the olive oil, the garlic, and the rice to a medium saucepan over medium-high heat and stir to combine. Add the water, sea salt, and black pepper and stir again. Once the water begins to boil, turn the heat down to low. Leave uncovered, stirring occasionally. When the water is nearly absorbed, about 25 to 30 minutes, add remaining ¼ cup of olive oil along with the chives, parsley, and basil. Stir until the herbs are incorporated and all the water is absorbed.

# SPEARMINT-PISTACHIO GELATO

GELATO REMINDS US OF romantic sidewalk strolls, cups in hand, sunshine on our faces. There's a slow pace to life when we find ourselves indulging in this Italian ice cream, so we think the preparation should feel the same: rhythmic, full, and meandering. Enjoy with a shot of espresso and someone you love.  SERVES 4

1 cup unsalted shelled pistachios, plus 2 tablespoons chopped, for garnish

½ cup raw cane sugar, divided

4 large egg yolks

2 cups whole milk

¼ cup chopped fresh spearmint, plus 1 tablespoon chopped, for garnish

## HOW WE CREATE

In a food processor, process the pistachios with ¼ cup of the sugar until the nuts are finely ground.

In a large bowl, whisk the egg yolks and the remaining ¼ cup sugar. Combine the pistachio mixture, milk, and spearmint in a medium saucepan over high heat and bring to a boil. Remove from the heat.

Gradually whisk the milk mixture, ¼ cup at a time, into the egg yolk mixture, stirring constantly and making sure the eggs do not begin to cook. Once combined, return the mixture to the saucepan. Stir over medium-low heat until it thickens, 7 to 8 minutes. Remove from the heat and transfer to a large heat-safe container.

Refrigerate until cold, about 3 hours. Remove the mixture from the fridge. If you prefer your gelato with a smooth consistency, strain the custard with a fine-mesh strainer. Pour the custard into an ice cream maker and follow the manufacturer's directions. Serve immediately, garnished with chopped pistachios and spearmint, or reserve in the freezer for a firmer consistency or later enjoyment.

> WELLNESS NOTE: Basic gelato recipes begin with egg yolks, sugar, and whole milk and integrate real foods like fresh fruit and nuts. It's a natural treat that makes for a special occasion.

# MASCARPONE AND HONEY STUFFED FIGS WITH A BALSAMIC REDUCTION

BALSAMIC VINEGAR IS ONE of those very versatile pantry essentials. Its robust aroma and bold flavor can bring life to a number of dishes, including healthy fruit-based desserts. When it's reduced, balsamic vinegar becomes a sweet, fermented grape syrup rather than a pungent acidic liquid. See page 58 to see how you can create a savory dish with melons, herbs, prosciutto, and balsamic reduction. SERVES 4

4 ounces mascarpone cheese

¼ cup chopped pecans

8 medium figs (any variety)

16 mint leaves

1 tablespoon minced fresh rosemary

4 teaspoons raw honey

1 tablespoon Balsamic Reduction (page 93)

½ teaspoon sea salt

## HOW WE CREATE

In a medium bowl, stir the mascarpone cheese and chopped pecans together.

Slice the figs in half and place each half on top of a mint leaf. Evenly spread mascarpone and pecan mixture on each fig half. Sprinkle the rosemary evenly on top of each fig. Drizzle with the honey and balsamic reduction, and finish with the salt.

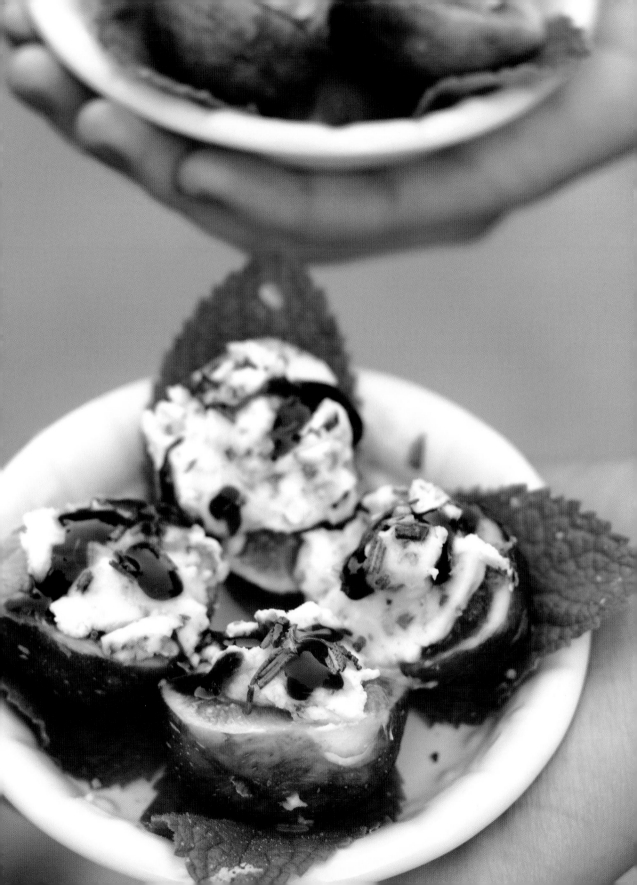

# HONEY-FIG JAM

FIGS ARE FOOD that fill the soul. Honey comes in at a close second. Simple as that.  MAKES 1½ CUPS

4 cups chopped figs

¼ cup raw honey

¼ cup water

1 tablespoon fresh lemon juice (about ½ small lemon)

½ teaspoon ground cinnamon

¼ teaspoon sea salt

## HOW WE CREATE

Combine ingredients in a medium saucepan and bring to a boil, stirring frequently. Reduce the heat to low and simmer until the mixture is thick, 15 to 20 minutes. Some chunks of figs may remain, and this is fine. Serve with an antipasto platter, crackers, or whole wheat toast. Store the remainder of the jam in a jar in the fridge for 4 to 6 weeks.

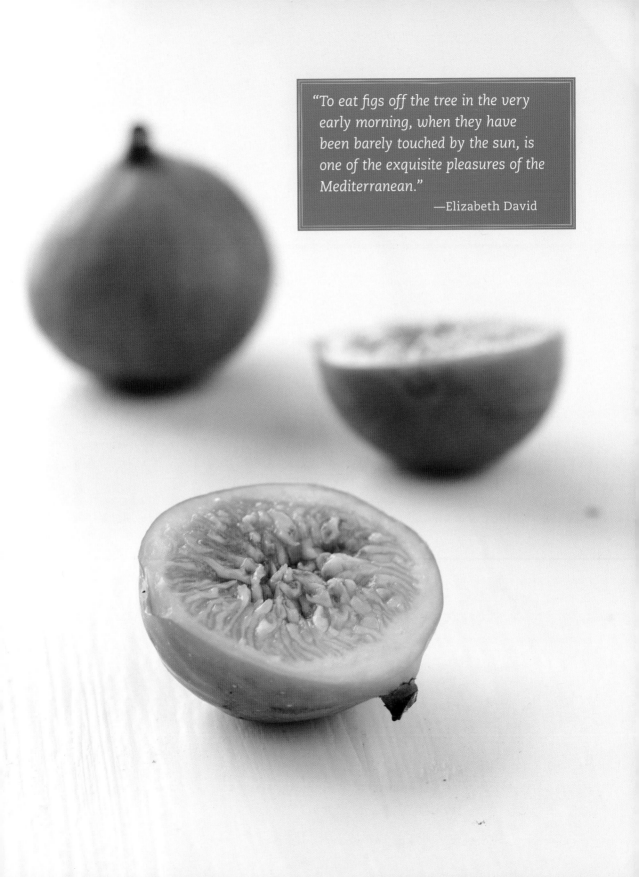

"To eat figs off the tree in the very early morning, when they have been barely touched by the sun, is one of the exquisite pleasures of the Mediterranean."

—Elizabeth David

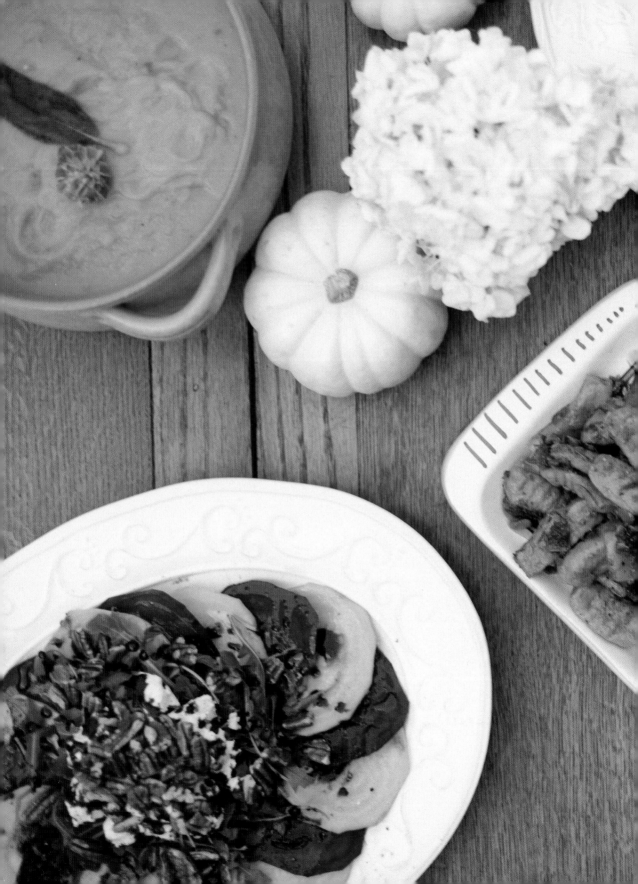

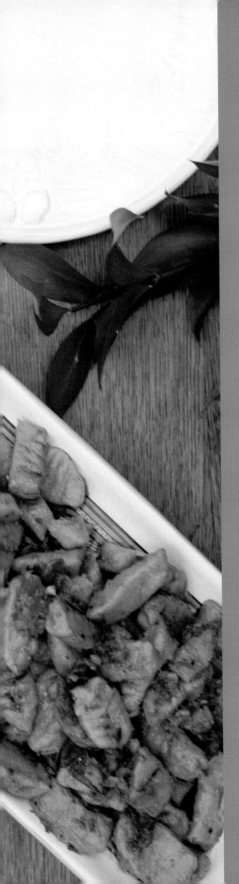

# AUTUMN

*"Give me juicy autumnal fruit, ripe and red from the orchard. Give me the splendid silent sun."*

—Walt Whitman

Autumn is just as much a state of mind as it is a change in the weather. The season brings a comforting feeling that accompanies a slower, kinder, and calmer pace of life. It brings to the table nutrient-dense foods like apples, pomegranates, tangerines, pears, winter squash, and sweet potatoes. We love the warmth that autumn brings—the soups, the sauces, the spices, and the smells.

# AVOCADO DEVILED EGGS

DEVILED EGGS ARE a popular European delicacy, dating all the way back to ancient Rome. For us, they date back to our childhood, as both of our grandmothers would feed us deviled eggs to hold us over before dinner. We put a spin on the classic deviled egg by cutting down on the yolk and adding avocado to maintain that creamy filling and that comforting feeling. MAKES 12 (SERVES 6)

6 eggs

1 large avocado

2 tablespoons minced parsley, plus
  leaves to garnish

½ cup minced red onion

1 garlic clove, minced

sea salt

black pepper

½ teaspoon red pepper flakes

## HOW WE CREATE

Place the eggs in a small saucepan and cover with cool water. Bring the water to a boil over medium heat. Once the boil is reached, turn off the burner and let the eggs sit for about 7 minutes, with the lid on, before running them under cool water. Peel the eggs and cut them in half lengthwise. Discard 3 of the yolks and spoon the remaining yolks into a mixing bowl. Add the avocado, parsley, onion, garlic, and salt and pepper, to taste. Mash with a fork until well combined and smooth the mixture with a spoon. Spoon the mixture back into the egg white halves and sprinkle the red pepper flakes evenly among them. Garnish each egg with a leaf or two of parsley before serving.

> WELLNESS NOTE: In combination, eggs and avocado are high in protein and heart-healthy fatty acids. Try spreading avocado and sliced hardboiled eggs, or these deviled eggs, on top of whole-grain toast for a power-packed breakfast.

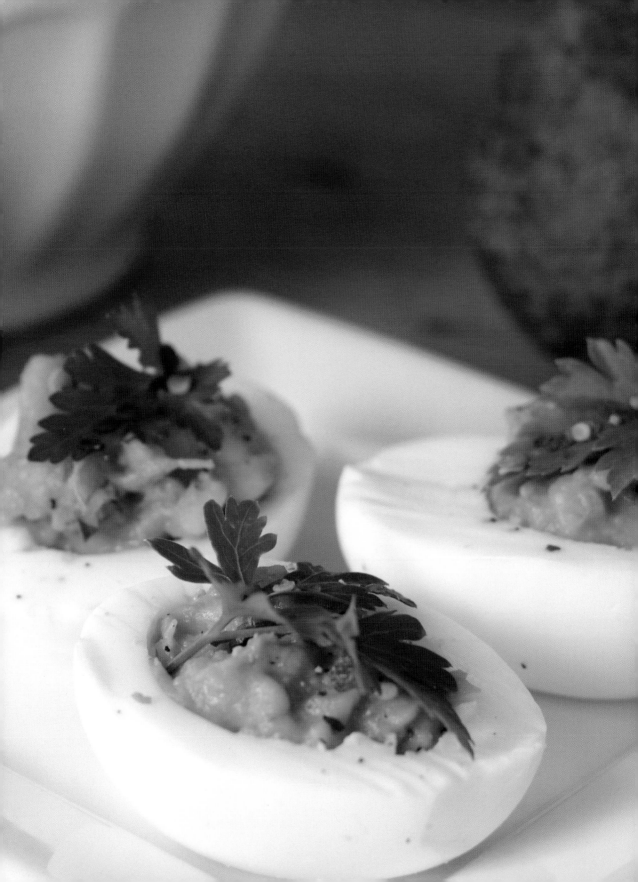

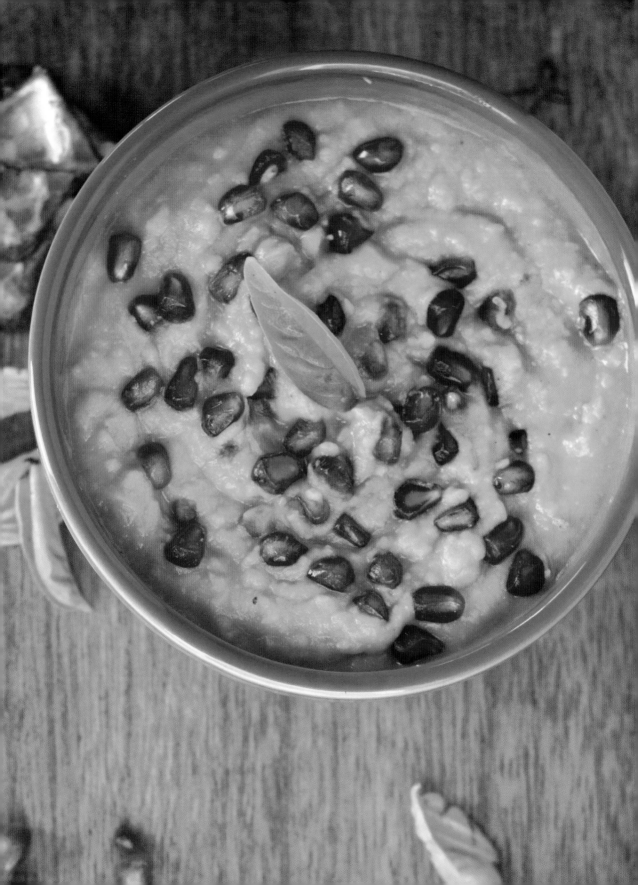

# BUTTERNUT SQUASH–POMEGRANATE HUMMUS

THIS RECIPE TAKES a traditional appetizer and gives it a modern autumn makeover. The hummus, with its seasonally spiced sweetness and vibrant pomegranates seeds, makes for a festive and healthy snack. These flavors make for a tasty soup (served hot or cold) as well—just cut the amount of garbanzo beans in half and follow the same steps. SERVES 8

1 medium butternut squash

2 tablespoons raw honey

2 tablespoons extra-virgin olive oil

1 garlic clove, minced

1 (15-ounce) can garbanzo beans, or 1½ cups home-cooked garbanzo beans

2 tablespoons fresh lemon juice (about 1 small lemon)

4 large basil leaves, plus more for garnish

½ teaspoon cayenne pepper

¼ cup pomegranate seeds

sea salt

black pepper

## HOW WE CREATE

Preheat the oven to 375º F.

Cut the butternut squash in half lengthwise and scoop out and discard the seeds. Drizzle with the olive oil and honey, and season with sea salt and black pepper. Top with the garlic. Place in the oven on a baking sheet, flesh-side up, and bake for about 45 minutes to an hour, or until tender.

Let the squash cool completely, then scoop the squash and garlic out with a spoon into a food processor or blender. Add the garbanzo beans, lemon juice, basil leaves, and cayenne pepper, and blend until smooth.

Transfer to a medium bowl and top with the pomegranate seeds and additional basil. Serve with whole wheat pita bread.

# RED WINE AND GARLIC STEAMED MUSSELS

MUSSELS HAVE AN ABILITY to jazz up even the most mundane of days. They're inexpensive, but fancy. We see them as a food that helps us with the transition from summer to fall: during the summer, we steam them in a white wine, and during the fall, we switch to red. We like to serve them alongside a simple lemon juice, fresh thyme, and olive oil pasta or with baked lemon and thyme mushrooms (as a crusty warm baguette goes well with both the mushrooms and the mussels). SERVES 4

1 tablespoon extra-virgin olive oil

3 large garlic cloves, minced

1 small sweet yellow onion, diced

2 celery stalks, chopped

2 medium tomatoes, chopped

½ teaspoon red pepper flakes (or more if you like it spicy)

¾ cup dry red wine

1 pound mussels, cleaned and debearded

1 handful fresh parsley, stems mostly removed (about 1 cup)

2 tablespoons chopped fresh basil

black pepper

## HOW WE CREATE

In a large skillet or saucepan, heat the olive oil over medium heat. Add the garlic, onion, and celery, and cook for about 4 minutes, stirring occasionally, until tender. Add the black pepper, tomatoes, red pepper flakes, and red wine. Stir again. Let simmer for about 5 minutes over medium-high heat. Add the mussels and cover with a lid, allowing the mussels to steam for about 7 minutes, or until they open. Add the parsley and basil. Remove from heat and discard any mussels that haven't opened. Serve and let mussel mayhem ensue.

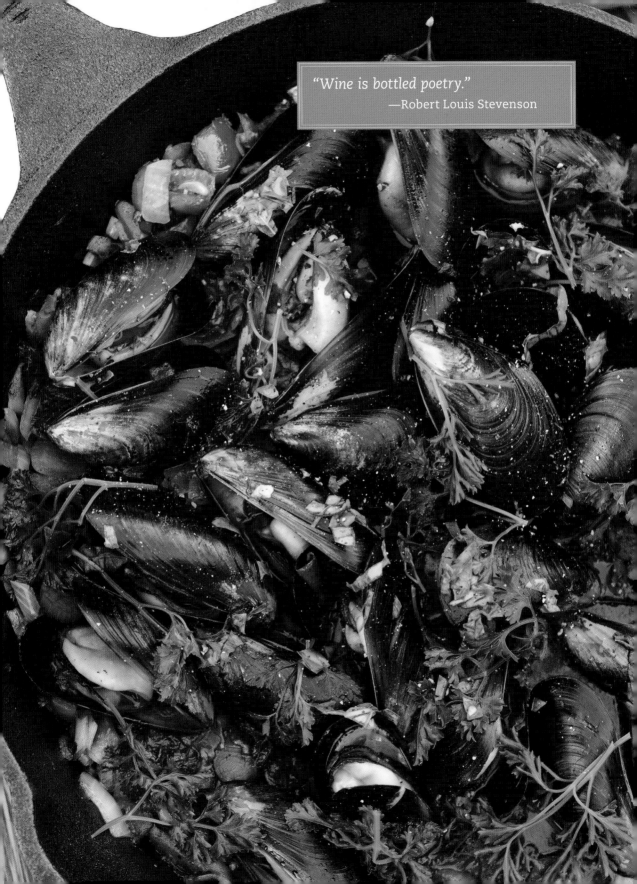

"Wine is bottled poetry."
—Robert Louis Stevenson

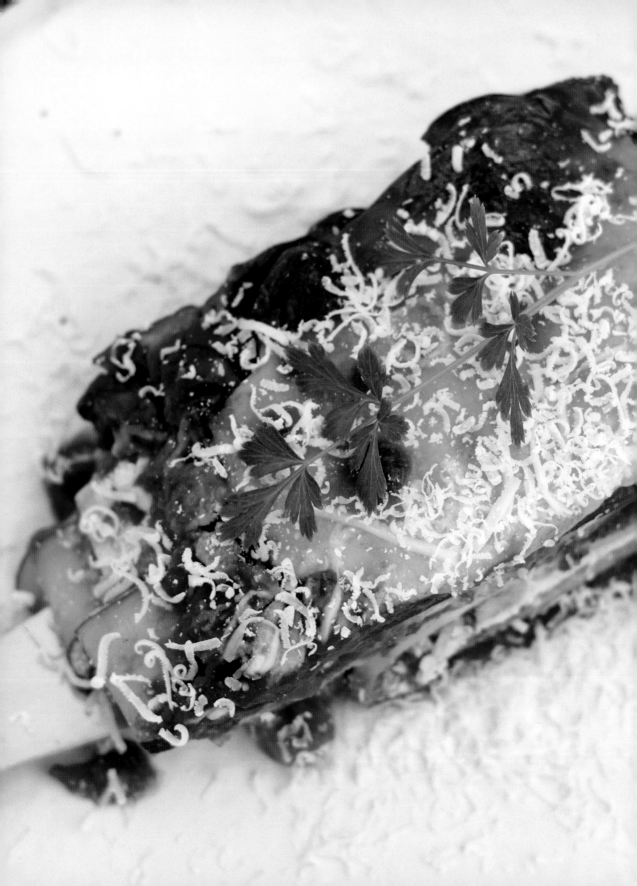

# ZUCCHINI LASAGNA

HOMEMADE LASAGNA is the kind of meal that makes you feel warm inside. We make it once or twice every few months with a Bolognese sauce, but this version of it is lighter, vegetarian, gluten-free, and definitely on the healthier side.  SERVES 8

## FOR THE MARINARA SAUCE

¼ cup extra-virgin olive oil

1 medium red onion, minced

2 celery stalks, minced

1 medium carrot, minced

½ fennel bulb, chopped

16 ounces (1 pound) cremini mushrooms, sliced

5 garlic cloves, minced

¼ cup dry red wine

1 (28-ounce) can San Marzano tomatoes

12 fresh basil leaves, chopped

12 fresh oregano leaves, chopped

3 whole bay leaves

¼ cup freshly grated Parmigiano-Reggiano cheese

sea salt

black pepper

## FOR THE LASAGNA

7 medium (about 2 pounds) zucchini, sliced into 1/8-inch strips

2 cups ricotta cheese

2 eggs

¼ teaspoon black pepper

1 tablespoon extra-virgin olive oil

¾ cup grated Parmigiano-Reggiano cheese

1 pound mozzarella cheese, sliced into ¼-inch-thick circles

½ tablespoon chopped fresh oregano

½ tablespoon chopped fresh parsley

## HOW WE CREATE

Preheat the oven to 350°F.

To make the sauce, in a large saucepan over medium heat, warm the olive oil and sauté the onion, celery, carrot, fennel, and a pinch of sea salt for 3 to 4 minutes, stirring occasionally. Stir in the mushrooms, then add the garlic and red wine and stir, scraping any vegetables that may be stuck to the bottom of the pan. Cover and let cook for about 3 minutes, allowing the flavors to blend. Then add the tomatoes, basil, oregano, bay leaves, a pinch or two of sea salt and some black pepper and stir. Reduce the heat to low and simmer for about 1½ hours uncovered to achieve the best flavor, stirring occasionally. When done, turn off the heat, add the Parmigiano-Reggiano, and stir until fully incorporated. Cover and set aside.

To make the lasagna, place your sliced zucchini on 2 large baking sheets lined with parchment paper or lightly coated with olive oil. Sprinkle with sea salt and roast for 10 to 15 minutes to dry the zucchini and decrease the natural moisture. Meanwhile, in a large bowl, combine the ricotta, eggs, and pepper. Stir until blended. Once zucchini is done, remove from the oven and let cool for about 10 minutes. Blot zucchini dry with paper towels to absorb any excess moisture.

Spread a light coat of olive oil on the bottom and sides of a 9 x 13-inch casserole dish to prevent sticking. Ladle in enough sauce to thinly cover the bottom of the pan and place a layer of zucchini slices over the sauce. Then, add enough sauce to cover the zucchini, and sprinkle some Parmigiano-Reggiano over it. Smooth half of the ricotta mixture into the dish, then top with another layer of zucchini. Spread another layer of sauce, then a layer of the mozzarella and Parmigiano-Reggiano. Repeat with another layer of zucchini, then sauce, and the rest of the ricotta, then finish with layers of zucchini, sauce, mozzarella, and Parmigiano-Reggiano until you reach the top of the pan, finishing with the Parmigiano-Reggiano. Top with the oregano and parsley.

Bake, covered with an aluminum foil "tent," leaving room for the cheese to melt untouched by the aluminum foil for 1 hour. Remove the foil tent and turn the oven to broil. Brown the top of the lasagna, 1 to 2 minutes depending on your broiler, but be careful not to burn the cheese. Remove and let cool for about 10 minutes, uncovered, before serving.

Leftover sauce and lasagna holds well in the freezer for 6 months or in the refrigerator for 1 week and can be easily reheated or eaten cold. Keep in mind, the layers of the zucchini lasagna may not hold together perfectly when freshly out of the oven.

# BARLEY RISOTTO WITH MUSHROOM, FIG, AND ARUGULA

TRADITIONALLY RISOTTO IS MADE with butter, but to follow the Mediterranean diet we use olive oil. The point is to coat each grain in a film of fat (called *tostatura*) and to then add the wine and allow the grains to absorb it. Risotto is also normally made with Arborio rice, but we found, after some experimentation, that whole-grain barley cooks up just as creamy.  SERVES 4

½ cup extra-virgin olive oil, divided

1 medium sweet yellow onion, minced

3 garlic cloves, minced

1½ cups sliced cremini mushrooms

1 cup chopped figs (any variety)

3 tablespoons chopped fresh parsley

1 cup hulled barley

1 teaspoon sea salt

½ cup dry white wine

1 bay leaf

4 cups vegetable broth

4 cups loosely packed baby arugula

½ cup freshly grated Parmigiano-Reggiano cheese

black pepper

## HOW WE CREATE

In a medium saucepan, heat the vegetable broth over medium heat for about 10 minutes, until hot.

In a large pot over medium heat, warm ¼ cup of the olive oil and sauté the onion for about 4 minutes, or until tender. Add the garlic, mushrooms, figs, and parsley, and sauté until tender, about 5 minutes. Add the barley, sea salt, and black pepper to taste, and stir to coat everything with oil. Add the white wine and bay leaf, and stir well. Add ½ cup of the hot vegetable broth, stirring constantly until all of the liquid has been absorbed. Continue to stir and add hot broth in small batches until the barley mixture is creamy and al dente. This may resemble a mini workout, as it takes 30 to 45 minutes. Remove from the heat, and stir in the remaining ¼ cup olive oil, along with the arugula and Parmigiano-Reggiano. Mix together until the arugula wilts, and serve immediately.

# GARLIC-HERB SPAGHETTI SQUASH WITH LEMON

THE OBLONG SPAGHETTI SQUASH is a truly magical food. Often when we eat pasta, we feel the need to combat the carbs with lots of veggies or a lean meat. Spaghetti squash gives us the same pasta-type feel, yet we love to mix it with nothing but the beautiful simplicity of fresh herbs, garlic, lemon juice, and olive oil. And of course, the Parmigiano-Reggiano is the final— and most important—ingredient to this lovely yellow treat. SERVES 4

1 large spaghetti squash

¼ cup extra-virgin olive oil, plus more for drizzling

3 large garlic cloves, minced

2 tablespoons minced fresh basil

1 teaspoon fresh thyme leaves

1 teaspoon minced fresh oregano

2 tablespoons fresh lemon juice (about 1 small lemon)

¼ cup shaved Parmigiano-Reggiano

black pepper

## HOW WE CREATE

Preheat the oven to 350°F.

Start by cutting the spaghetti squash in half. Spaghetti squash is notoriously difficult to cut, and there are numerous ways to do it. Some swear by placing it on the counter and hacking it in half with a sharp butcher knife. Others cut off both ends and slice the squash while it's standing. We use a sharp serrated knife and take our time rocking the knife in and out, leaving the stem on so as to use the hollowed-out squash as a bowl.

Regardless of how you get there, once your squash is in half, scoop out the seeds and discard them. Drizzle the inside with olive oil and season with sea salt and black pepper. Place skin-side up on a baking sheet, and bake in the oven for 35 minutes. Remove from the oven, flip the halves over so that the flesh can breathe, and let cool for about 15 minutes. Once cool, use a fork to scrape the squash strands out, as if scooping. Set aside on a large plate or flat surface.

Heat the ¼ cup olive oil in a large skillet over medium heat. Add the garlic, basil, thyme, oregano, spaghetti squash, and lemon juice all together. Sauté for about 10 minutes, or until the ingredients are fully incorporated. Remove from the heat and garnish with black pepper and shaved Parmigiano-Reggiano.

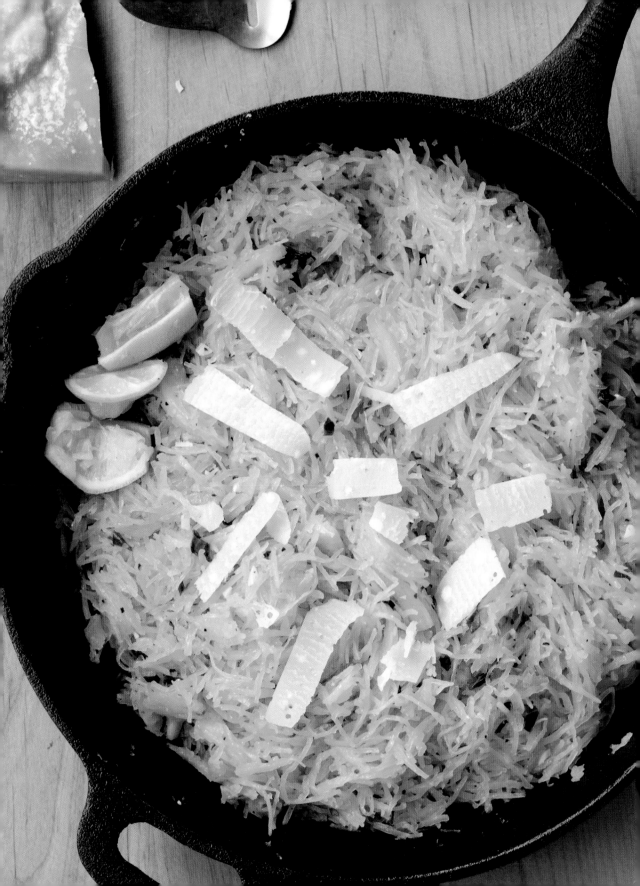

# SWEET POTATO GNOCCHI WITH HONEY CRISP APPLES

THOUGH THIS RECIPE REQUIRES you set aside some time in the kitchen, the end result is rich, decadent and oh-so-very rewarding. Our favorite thing about this dish is that it is simultaneously sweet and savory, and goes well with a simple spinach or arugula salad or roasted asparagus spears. SERVES 4

## FOR THE GNOCCHI

2 pounds sweet potatoes

¾ cup whole wheat flour

¾ cup unbleached all-purpose flour

1 egg yolk

⅛ teaspoon ground nutmeg

1 teaspoon sea salt, plus more for the water

## FOR THE SAUCE

¾ cup extra-virgin olive oil, divided

4 large garlic cloves, sliced

2 Honey Crisp apples, chopped

1 cup chopped sweet potato skins

2 tablespoons chopped fresh rosemary

2 tablespoons chopped fresh basil

1 tablespoon chopped fresh oregano

2 tablespoons raw honey

½ teaspoon ground cinnamon

sea salt

black pepper

¼ cup shaved Parmigiano-Reggiano cheese

## HOW WE CREATE

To make the gnocchi, boil the sweet potatoes for about 40 minutes, until they can be easily pierced with a fork. When cool enough to handle, peel, reserving the peels, and pass the potatoes through a ricer.

Place the riced potatoes in a large skillet over medium heat. Cook for 10 minutes, or until some of the liquid has cooked off. The more liquid that evaporates, the fluffier your gnocchi will be. Spread the mash across the pan to expose as much of its surface as possible to cool.

In a medium bowl, whisk together the whole wheat flour and all-purpose flour. On a lightly floured surface, gather the cooled sweet potato mash into a mound and form a well in the center with your hands. Add the egg yolk to the well, and sprinkle ½ cup of the flour mixture, along with the nutmeg and sea salt over the entire mound. Work everything together with your hands. Add flour little by little until the dough becomes a ball. This should take about all the flour, 1½ cups total. Cut the dough into 4 equal parts.

Sprinkle flour on your work surface and the dough. Flour your hands. Roll each piece of dough into a rope about ½ inch thick. Slice each rope into ½-inch pieces. Use a fork to create ribs along each dumpling (this will allow the sauce to stick to the dumplings).

Bring a large pot of heavily salted water to a boil (about 2 tablespoons sea salt to 6 quarts of water). In batches of 10 to 12, drop the gnocchi into the water, stirring gently and continuously, until they rise to the surface, 2 to 3 minutes. As each batch is finished, transfer the cooked dumplings to a large baking pan and keep covered with aluminum foil. When all of the dumplings are cooked, hold them warm under the foil while you prepare the sauce. Transfer them to the skillet with the sauce.

To make the sauce, in a large skillet over medium-high heat, warm ¼ cup of the olive oil and the garlic. When the garlic begins to sizzle, add the apples, potato skins, rosemary, basil, oregano, honey, cinnamon, and sea salt. Stir frequently until the potato skins begin to crisp. Add the dumplings and black pepper to the skillet, and pour in the remaining ½ cup olive oil. Stir until fully coated. Serve topped with shaved Parmigiano-Reggiano.

WELLNESS NOTE: We eat sweet potatoes regularly as a breakfast hash with veggies or in scrambled eggs, baked as chips with some olive oil and cinnamon, or mashed and served with chicken. They are inexpensive, delicious, and full of vitamins.

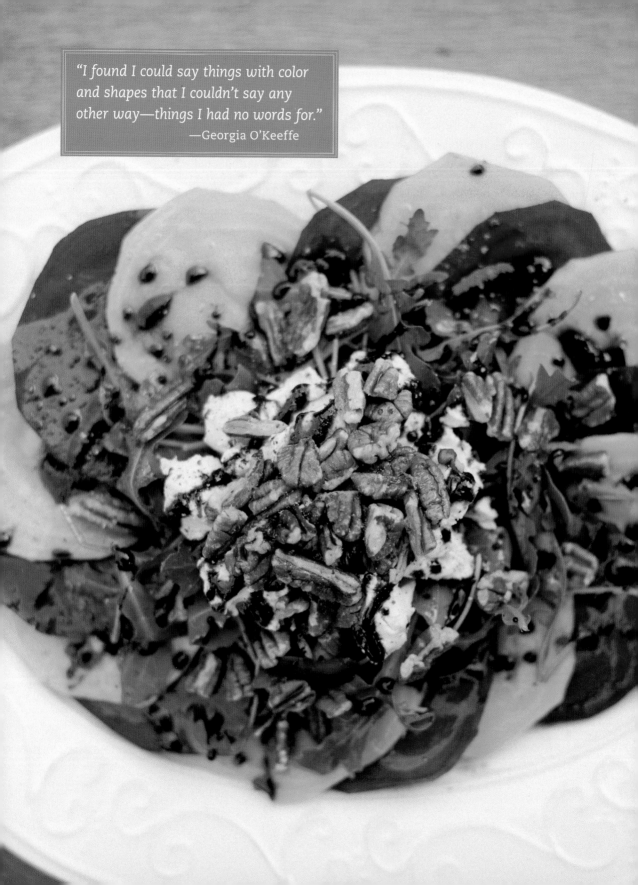

"I found I could say things with color and shapes that I couldn't say any other way—things I had no words for."
—Georgia O'Keeffe

# BEET CARPACCIO

WE LOVE THE COLORS, shapes, and tastes of this dish, and no matter how many times we eat it, it always feels like a delicacy. Don't discard your beet greens, as they contain a plethora of health benefits and even contain more iron than spinach does. Instead, prepare them in the same way that you would prepare Swiss chard or rapini (pages 47 and 96). May this salad inspire you to make beet art! SERVES 4

½ cup balsamic vinegar

2 medium beets (golden, red, or Chioggia, if available)

1 cup arugula

4 ounces goat cheese

¼ cup chopped walnuts or pecans

2 tablespoons extra-virgin olive oil

sea salt

black pepper

## HOW WE CREATE

Begin by making the balsamic vinegar reduction, which sounds intimidating to some, but couldn't be easier. Pour the balsamic into a small saucepan over medium-high heat and cook for 5 to 10 minutes, or until it thickens like a glaze. It should reduce by about half. Try not to bring it to a complete boil. Remove the glaze from the heat and allow it to cool. Set aside.

Peel and slice the beets into thin circles using a sharp knife or mandolin. Arrange them on a plate in a circle, alternating between the colors. Place the arugula in the center of the circle and top with the goat cheese and walnuts or pecans. Drizzle the balsamic reduction and the olive oil over the salad. Season with sea salt and black pepper.

# WHOLE ROASTED APPLE-ROSEMARY CHICKEN

IN THIS RECIPE, the assertive and piney flavor of fresh rosemary blends well with the richness of the balsamic vinegar and the sweetness of the apples. Your classic weeknight chicken meal now boasts an entirely new array of flavors. If it's a warm autumn evening and you're feeling adventurous, you can also feel free to throw this on the grill (which is what we usually do). SERVES 4 TO 6 (PERHAPS WITH LEFTOVERS)

1 apple, seeded and quartered (any variety)

4 tablespoons extra-virgin olive oil, divided

4 tablespoons balsamic vinegar, divided

4 tablespoons fresh rosemary leaves, divided

1 (3- to 4-pound) whole chicken, giblets removed

1 lemon, halved

sea salt

black pepper

## HOW WE CREATE

Preheat the oven to 425°F.

In a small bowl, mix the apple slices with 2 tablespoons of the oil, 2 tablespoons of the balsamic vinegar, and 2 tablespoons of the rosemary. Season with sea salt and black pepper to taste. Toss lightly. Place the chicken in a roasting pan and stuff with the apple mixture. Drizzle with the remaining balsamic and olive oil, top with the remaining rosemary, and season with sea salt and black pepper. Squeeze the two lemon halves over the chicken and lay the leftover lemon halves on each chicken leg. Roast for about 45 minutes. Remove the chicken, and let cool for about 15 minutes before slicing.

# PEAR AND PROSECCO TILAPIA

ALTHOUGH THIS MEAL may sound fancy, it's incredibly easy to throw together. This dish is great with Garlic-Herb Rice (page 70), and/or any simple salad or green leaf sauté. The flavors of pear, prosecco, and lemon juice not only make a tasty fish dish, they also make for a light soup when combined with fish or vegetable stock.

For a special touch, enjoy your remaining prosecco with a few pomegranate seeds or pieces of sliced pear thrown into a champagne flute.  SERVES 4

¼ cup extra-virgin olive oil

3 large garlic cloves, minced

3 medium pears, sliced flat, about ¼ inch thick

8 large whole basil leaves, plus more for garnish

⅓ cup prosecco

4 (4- to 6-ounce) tilapia fillets

2 tablespoons fresh lemon juice (about 1 small lemon)

sea salt

black pepper

thin lemon slices, for garnish

## HOW WE CREATE

Warm the olive oil over medium-high heat in a medium skillet. Add the garlic, pears, and basil leaves, and pour in the prosecco. While the ingredients begin to sizzle, lay the tilapia over the pears, and then top with lemon juice, sea salt, and black pepper. Cover the skillet with a lid and let cook for about 4 minutes. Remove the lid and flip the fish to cook for another 4 minutes, making sure to gently mix the other ingredients while doing so. The fish is done when it flakes with a fork.

Serve the tilapia over the sautéed ingredients and top with basil, black pepper, and a sliver of lemon for garnish.

# SIMPLE SAUTÉED RAPINI

NICK'S GRANDFATHER (PAPA) used to come home with huge, luscious bunches of rapini in hand, picked fresh from wild fields near his home and wrapped in newspaper. Rapini is actually a descendant of the turnip tribe, and while some people love it, others definitely do not. It's extremely bitter, but when it's cooked correctly, it can become a simple masterpiece. It pairs beautifully with heartier dishes like roast chicken, spaghetti and meatballs, and potatoes. SERVES 4

¼ cup extra-virgin olive oil

5 large garlic cloves, chopped

1 medium red onion, roughly chopped

2 bunches rapini, 2 inches of stem trimmed off

½ teaspoon red pepper flakes (optional)

sea salt

black pepper

## HOW WE CREATE

In a large skillet, heat the olive oil and add garlic and onion, cooking over medium heat for 3 to 4 minutes, until onions are tender, stirring frequently. Add the rapini and red pepper flakes, and season with sea salt and black pepper. Stir to combine. Cover with a lid and cook for about 7 minutes. Uncover and stir frequently, sautéing for about 3 more minutes.

# MINT-CARROT CABBAGE WEDGE

THE LEMON JUICE will seep into the crevices of this cabbage wedge salad to surprise and awaken your tastes buds to the rest of your meal's flavors. It's the perfect crispy and colorful accompaniment to the texture and simplicity of a dense and clean fish, like the halibut on page 65.  SERVES 4

½ head purple cabbage

½ cup extra-virgin olive oil

2 tablespoons fresh lemon juice (about 1 small lemon)

2 carrots, shredded (we like to use rainbow carrots)

12 mint leaves, chopped

sea salt

black pepper

## HOW WE CREATE

Cut the cabbage into quarters to make 4 wedge slices.

Mix the olive oil and lemon juice in a small bowl, and season to taste with sea salt and black pepper. On four separate plates, place equal amounts of shredded carrots and place a cabbage wedges on top of each one. Garnish with mint, drizzle with dressing, and enjoy.

# BAKED LEMON AND
# THYME MUSHROOMS

THERE'S SOMETHING ENTICING about warm mushrooms, softly cooked and enveloped in a blanket of tangy citrus juices and Parmigiano-Reggiano. We eat this alongside a thick loaf of bread and tear, dip, eat, and repeat.  SERVES 4

grated zest of 1 lemon

3 tablespoons chopped fresh thyme (preferably lemon thyme)

1 garlic clove, minced

½ cup extra-virgin olive oil

2 pounds cremini mushrooms, cleaned and sliced

3 tablespoons fresh lemon juice (about 1½ lemons)

⅓ cup grated Parmigiano-Reggiano cheese

sea salt

black pepper

## HOW WE CREATE

Preheat the oven to 425°F.

In a small bowl, combine the lemon zest, thyme, garlic, and olive oil. Place the mushrooms in a single layer on a baking sheet and drizzle the oil mixture over them. Mix gently. Season with salt and pepper. Bake for 7 minutes. Stir and add the lemon juice and Parmigiano-Reggiano. Bake for another 4 to 5 minutes, or until cheese is golden. Serve with bread, simple pasta, or rice.

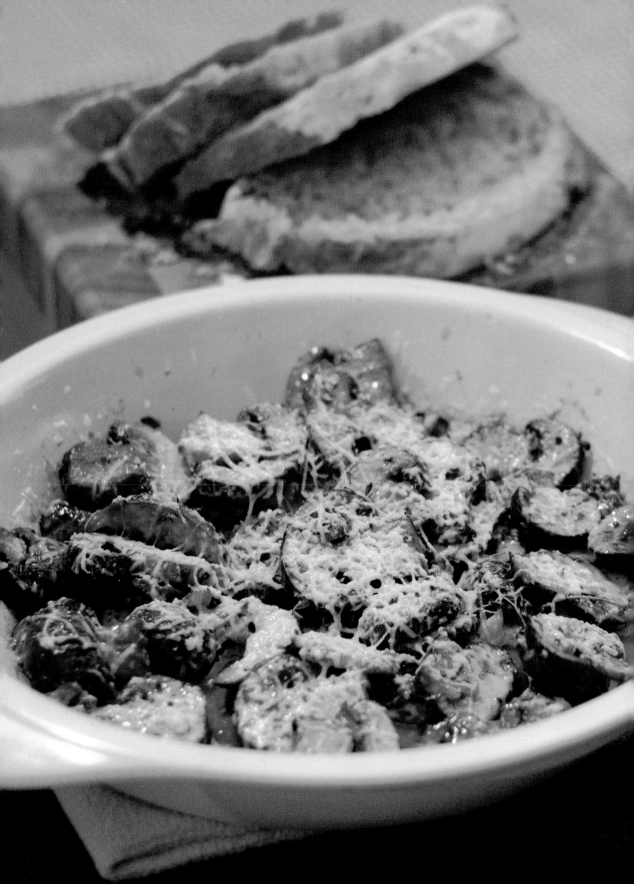

# ROASTED PUMPKIN APPLE SAGE SOUP

IN AUTUMN, THE OPTIONS for pumpkin dishes are endless—from ravioli and pie to breads, oatmeals, and soups. This is a simple, festive soup that leaves the sweet scent of fall wafting through the kitchen. It has become a tradition for us to prepare this every fall for large gatherings and we like to pack any leftovers we may have in a thermos for a crisp picnic under our favorite trees.  SERVES 6 TO 8

2 small or medium sugar pie pumpkins (about 6 pounds total)

½ cup extra-virgin olive oil

2 large garlic cloves, minced

1 small sweet yellow onion, finely chopped

3 apples (like Honey Crisp or Pink Lady), minced with skin on

2 tablespoons chopped fresh sage, plus whole leaves for garnish

5 cups low-sodium vegetable stock

sea salt

black pepper

## HOW WE CREATE

Preheat the oven to 425°F.

Cut the pumpkins in half using a sharp knife. Scoop out and discard the seeds. Place the pumpkins on a baking sheet, skin-side down, and bake for about 1 hour, until the flesh is tender and easy to scoop. Remove from the oven and let cool completely. Scoop out the flesh with a large spoon, yielding about 5 cups.

In a large pot, heat the olive oil over medium heat. Add the garlic, onion, apples, and sage, and sauté for about 4 minutes, until onion and apples are tender. Add the pumpkin, broth, salt, and pepper to the pot. Bring to a boil. Reduce the heat to low. Cover and simmer for 12 to 15 minutes to allow flavors to combine. Transfer to a blender or use an immersion blender, and blend until the soup is a smooth consistency. To serve, garnish each bowl with a leaf of fresh sage or, as we do, an edible flower.

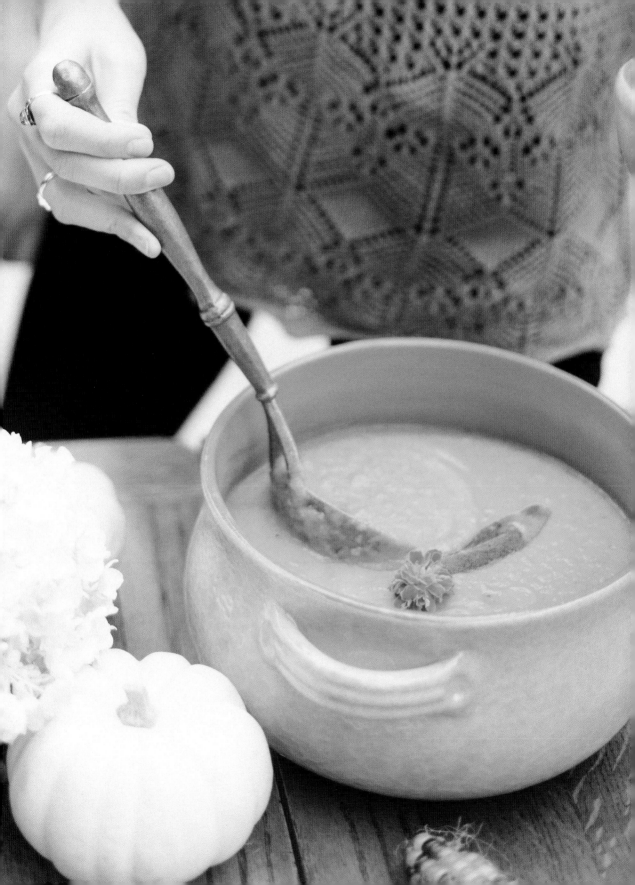

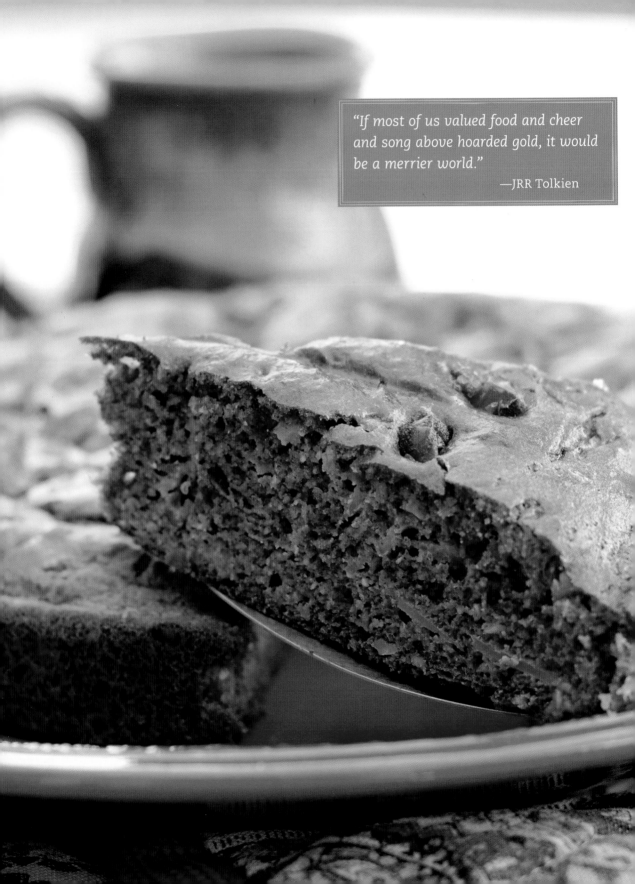

"If most of us valued food and cheer and song above hoarded gold, it would be a merrier world."

—JRR Tolkien

# ALMOND FLOUR ZUCCHINI-CARROT BREAKFAST CAKE

WE ONCE VENTURED TO Bay's aunt's whimsical storybook home in Ojai, California, after being on the road for a month. Following an evening of stories, pesto pasta, and plum tarts, we awoke the next morning to a healthy breakfast bread made with zucchini and carrots. Aunt Sissy calls it her "morning glory bread," and we were blown away by how tasty it was. Today, our own rendition of it makes its way to our kitchen quite frequently, as it takes all but 10 minutes to throw the ingredients together.  MAKES 1 (8-INCH) CAKE (SERVES 8)

2 cups almond flour

½ teaspoon ground nutmeg

2 ½ teaspoons ground cinnamon

1 teaspoon baking soda

½ teaspoon sea salt

3 eggs, beaten

¼ cup raw honey

1 tablespoon extra-virgin olive oil

1 ripe banana, mashed

½ cup shredded zucchini, unpeeled

½ cup shredded carrots

3 tablespoons chopped dates

## HOW WE CREATE

Preheat oven to 350°F. Lightly coat an 8-inch cake pan with olive oil.

In a medium bowl, combine the almond flour, nutmeg, cinnamon, baking soda, and sea salt, and set aside. In a large bowl, combine the eggs, honey, and olive oil. Fold in the banana, zucchini, carrots, and dates. Gradually add the dry mixture into the wet mixture, gently stirring to combine.

Pour the batter into the prepared pan. Bake for 30 to 35 minutes, until a toothpick inserted in the center comes out clean.

Drizzle honey on top for a little extra sweetness and serve it alongside Greek yogurt and berries. Aunt Sissy adds fresh orange juice and zest to her Greek yogurt, another creative tidbit we have learned over shared breakfasts.

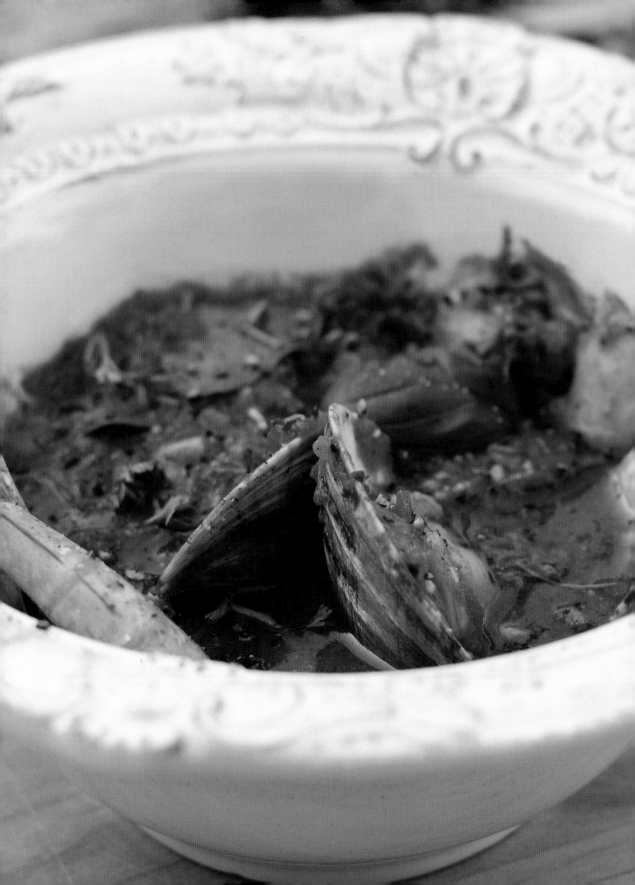

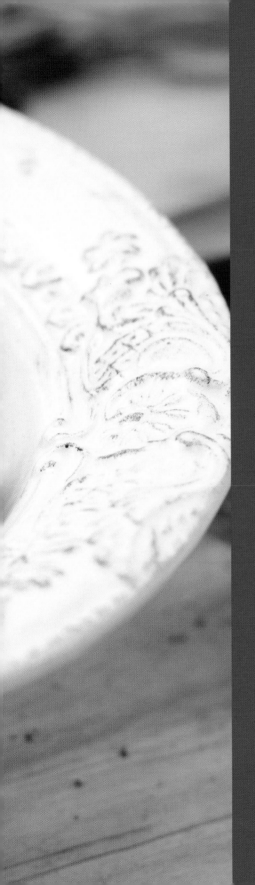

# WINTER

*You can't get too much winter in the winter.*

—Robert Frost

No matter where you are in the world—whether you are experiencing sunny days or snow storms—winter is a time of discovery, acceptance, and preparation for the following year. Vegetables like endives, broccoli, brussels sprouts, chicory, kale, fennel, and cauliflower are plentiful at this time, and it's a good season for flipping through cookbooks and taking a little extra time to stay home, relax, and prepare a meal. From soups to pastas to warm garlic sauces, our hope is that these meals keep you warm and help you to find what the Italians call *Il dolce far niente*—the sweetness of doing nothing.

# WARM ROSEMARY OLIVES

IT'S NOT UNCOMMON to walk into an Italian household and find a predinner snack of olives, carrots, celery, and fennel. During the winter, there's nothing like a plump warm olive with a fresh whole-grain baguette to absorb the juices of leftover oils and vinegar. Put out with a bowl of accompanying olive oil, a drizzle of balsamic, freshly chopped rosemary, ground black pepper, and some garlic to accompany these traditional flavors. SERVES 4

1 tablespoon extra-virgin olive oil

6 whole garlic cloves

1 large fennel bulb, sliced into ½- to 1-inch slices

2 large sprigs fresh rosemary

2 cups mixed whole, unpitted olives (like Greek, nicoise, and green)

½ teaspoon red pepper flakes

½ teaspoon black pepper

2 cups arugula

## HOW WE CREATE

In a large skillet on medium heat, warm the olive oil, add garlic and fennel, and sauté for about 4 minutes, until the fennel is tender. Take the rosemary leaves off of each sprig and throw them into the skillet along with the olives, red pepper flakes, and black pepper. Cook for 7 minutes, stirring occasionally. Turn off the heat and fold in the arugula. Transfer to a bowl and serve.

# TUSCAN TOMATO AND CANNELLINI BEAN SOUP WITH KALE

OUR FAVORITE THING about soup is that it's simple and homey. We add the ingredients, let them simmer, and then saunter off to a cozy corner to read a book or sip some tea. It's the kind of food that feels as good to make as it does to eat.  SERVES 4

2 tablespoons extra-virgin olive oil, plus more for garnish

1 medium red onion, minced

7 garlic cloves, minced

½ medium fennel bulb, chopped

2 teaspoons chopped fresh rosemary

4 cups vegetable stock

1 (14-ounce) can San Marzano tomatoes

2 (15-ounce) cans cannellini beans, or 3 cups home-cooked cannellini beans

1 tablespoon raw honey

1 teaspoon red pepper flakes

2 tablespoons chopped fresh parsley, plus more for garnish

5 cups chopped kale

¼ cup freshly grated Parmigiano-Reggiano cheese

sea salt

black pepper

## HOW WE CREATE

Heat the olive oil in a large saucepan over medium heat. Cook the onion, garlic, fennel, and rosemary for 5 minutes, stirring occasionally. Add the vegetable stock, tomatoes, beans, honey, red pepper flakes, and parsley, and season with sea salt and pepper to taste. Reduce the heat to low and simmer, uncovered, for 30 minutes, stirring occasionally. Stir in the kale and Parmigiano-Reggiano.

Transfer to four soup bowls. Garnish with fresh parsley, black pepper, sea salt, and a drizzle of olive oil.

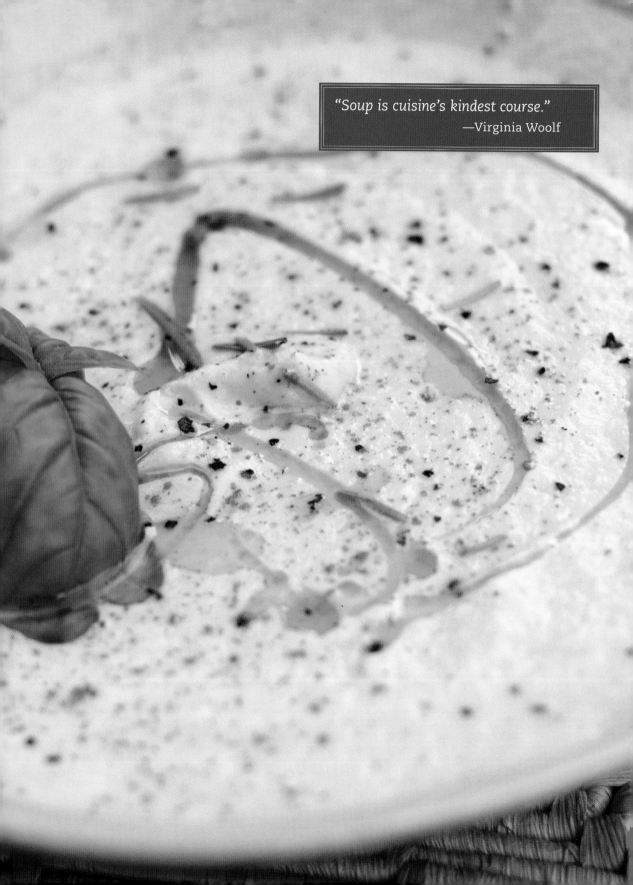

# ROASTED FENNEL AND CAULIFLOWER SOUP

ALTHOUGH THEY CAN BE found year round, fennel and cauliflower are by nature cool-weather crops, which makes them excellent ingredients for this healthy winter soup. This is a surprisingly filling dish, so we serve it as a main course rather than a starter (though you could cut the recipe in half and serve it before dinner as well).  SERVES 8

1 large fennel bulb, chopped (about 2 cups)

1 large head cauliflower, chopped (about 4 cups)

1 medium yellow onion, chopped, divided

4 tablespoons extra-virgin olive oil, divided, plus more for garnish

½ tablespoon raw honey

4 garlic cloves

2 tablespoons minced rosemary, plus more for garnish

⅓ cup packed fresh basil, plus more for garnish

2 cups water, plus more as needed

½ cup plain whole milk Greek yogurt

sea salt

black pepper

## HOW WE CREATE

Preheat the oven to 400°F.

Place the fennel, cauliflower, and half of the chopped onion onto a baking sheet and drizzle with 2 tablespoons of the olive oil and the honey, and sprinkle with salt and pepper. Roast for 20 minutes, or until tender. Remove from the oven.

After the veggies have roasted, add the remaining 2 tablespoons of olive oil to a large pot over medium heat and add the garlic cloves and the rest of the onion. Sauté for 4 minutes, until onions are tender. Add the roasted vegetables, rosemary, basil, and water, and cover and simmer on low for 30 to 45 minutes, until vegetables are soft, stirring occasionally.

Transfer to a food processor and add the Greek yogurt. Blend until smooth, and add more water 1 tablespoon at a time if it's too thick.

Transfer to bowls and garnish with olive oil, basil, and rosemary.

# CIOPPINO

ORIGINALLY SAID TO HAVE been made on boats by Italian fishermen while out at sea, cioppino is a fish stew that became popular in San Francisco in the 1800s. You'll often see it served with crab legs on top, and although this particular recipe doesn't call for that, you can feel free to get creative. Add a few things. Subtract a few things. You know the drill.  SERVES 4 TO 6

¼ cup extra-virgin olive oil

1 small sweet yellow onion, minced

½ cup minced fennel

5 garlic cloves, minced

4 (3-inch) anchovies, chopped, or ⅓ cup chopped sardines

1 teaspoon minced fresh thyme

1 tablespoon minced fresh oregano

½ tablespoon chopped fresh parsley

½ cup dry red wine

1 (28-ounce) can chopped San Marzano tomatoes

2 cups vegetable broth

2 whole bay leaves

pinch of sea salt

½ teaspoon red pepper flakes

1 pound skinless white fish fillets (like cod, red snapper, or halibut)

½ pound clams

½ pound large raw shrimp

4 to 6 basil leaves, for garnish

black pepper

## HOW WE CREATE

In a large pot, heat the olive oil over medium-high heat. Add the onion and fennel and sauté for 3 minutes. Add the garlic and anchovies or sardines, and stir until the ingredients are incorporated. Then add the thyme, oregano, parsley, and red wine, scraping up anything that is stuck to the pan with a wooden spoon. Pour in the tomatoes and vegetable broth, stir, and add the bay leaves, a pinch of sea salt, and the red pepper flakes. Bring the temperature down to low and simmer. Cover with the lid slightly open, stirring occasionally, for about 45 minutes. Uncover and stir in the fish fillets, leaving uncovered to cook for about 10 minutes, until fish begins to flake apart. Add the clams and shrimp, and let cook for about 7 to 10 minutes, until clams open, discarding any that remain closed. Taste and add sea salt if needed or more red pepper flakes for extra spice. Serve immediately, garnished with fresh black pepper and a basil leaf for each bowl.

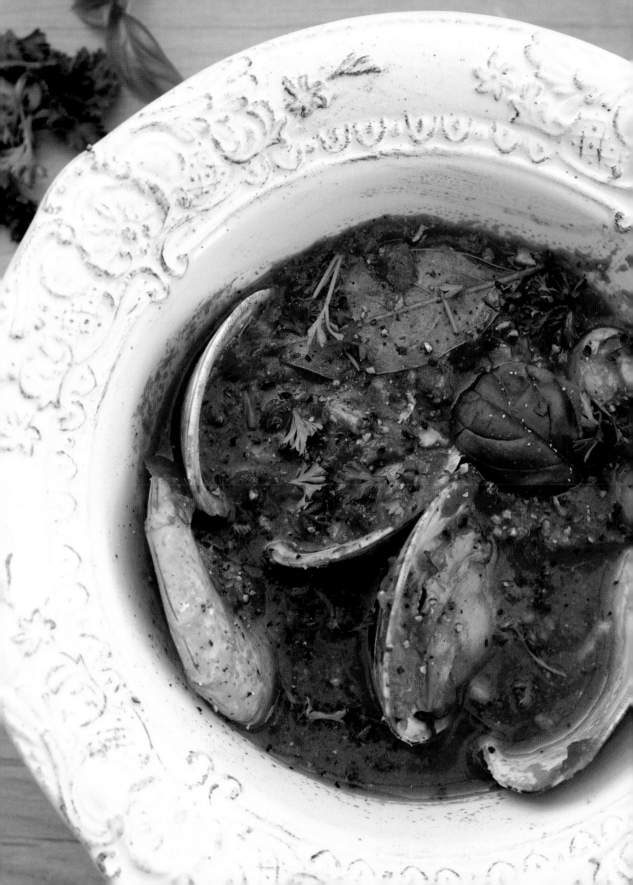

# SPAGHETTI AND TURKEY MEATBALLS

MUSHROOMS REPLACE BREAD CRUMBS and ground turkey is used in place of ground beef in this healthier alternative to the famous comfort food that is spaghetti and meatballs. SERVES 4

## FOR THE MEATBALLS

1 tablespoon extra-virgin olive oil

1 pound lean ground turkey

8 ounces cremini mushrooms, finely minced

1 egg, lightly beaten

3 garlic cloves, finely minced

¼ cup finely minced red onion

1 tablespoon chopped fresh parsley

1 tablespoon freshly grated Parmigiano-Reggiano cheese

1 teaspoon black pepper

1 teaspoon sea salt

## FOR THE MARINARA SAUCE

¼ cup extra-virgin olive oil

1 medium red onion, minced

2 celery stalks, minced

1 medium carrot, minced

5 garlic cloves, minced

¼ cup dry red wine

2 (28-ounce) cans San Marzano tomatoes

12 fresh basil leaves, chopped

12 fresh oregano leaves, chopped

3 whole bay leaves

sea salt

black pepper

¼ cup freshly grated Parmigiano-Reggiano cheese

## FOR THE PASTA

1 pound Spaghetti Fresh Pasta Dough (page 131)

## HOW WE CREATE

In a large bowl, use your hands to mix together all of the ingredients for the meatballs. When mixed well, begin to roll into balls of your desired size, making sure they are rolled nice and tightly so they stay together. Set aside on a baking sheet or plate lined with parchment paper.

To make the sauce, in a large saucepan over medium heat, warm the olive oil and sauté the red onion, celery, carrot, and a pinch of sea salt for 3 to 4 minutes, until ingredients begin to soften, stirring occasionally. Add the meatballs and sear until they begin to brown, then add the garlic and red wine and stir, scraping up any vegetables that may be stuck to the bottom of the pot.

Cover and let cook for about 3 minutes. Next, add the tomatoes, basil, oregano, and bay leaves, and season with sea salt and black pepper. Stir. Reduce the heat to low and simmer everything for up to 1½ hours, uncovered, to achieve the best flavor (making sure meatballs do not fall apart). When done, turn off the heat and add the Parmigiano-Reggiano. Stir until blended. Add to the cooked pasta in a large serving bowl. Toss lightly and enjoy.

Alternatively, if you are making a larger quantity of meatballs, you can bake them at 350°F (rather than sauté them in the pot) for about 25 minutes, or until browned. Add the meatballs to the sauce right after you add the tomatoes and herbs and allow them to simmer.

# CHICKEN SAUSAGE BARLEY RISOTTO
## WITH RAPINI AND SUN-DRIED TOMATOES

LIKE WITH THE BARLEY RISOTTO with Mushroom, Fig, and Arugula on page 87, here we substitute barley for the classic Aborio rice. Risotto works as a base with all sorts of vegetables, but we sure do love our rapini. For a healthier option, substitute 1 pound of chopped chicken breast for the sausage; if you do this, we suggest doubling the amount of herbs used and adding a touch of sea salt. SERVES 4

4 cups chicken broth

¼ cup extra-virgin olive oil

1 pound uncooked Italian chicken sausage, chopped

6 garlic cloves, minced

1 large bunch rapini, chopped

¼ cup chopped sun-dried tomatoes

1 cup hulled barley

1 tablespoon chopped fresh parsley

1 tablespoon chopped fresh basil

½ teaspoon red pepper flakes

¼ teaspoon fennel seeds

¼ cup chardonnay

½ cup shaved Manchego cheese

black pepper

## HOW WE CREATE

In a medium saucepan, heat the chicken stock over medium heat. In a large pot over medium heat, warm the olive oil and sauté the chicken sausage for about 4 minutes, until it begins to lightly brown. Add the garlic, rapini, and sun-dried tomatoes, and sauté for about 5 minutes, until rapini begins to soften. Add the barley, parsley, basil, red pepper flakes, fennel seeds, black pepper, to taste, and chardonnay, and stir. Add ½ cup of the hot chicken stock, stirring constantly until all of the liquid has been absorbed. Continue to stir and add hot stock in small amounts until the barley mixture is creamy and al dente. Remove from the heat, add the Manchego cheese and black pepper to taste, and serve immediately.

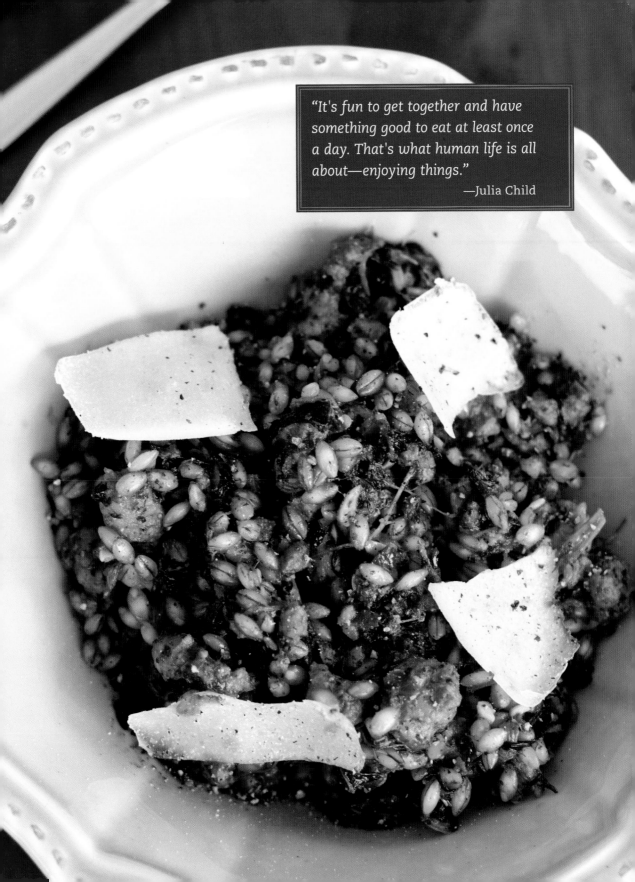

"It's fun to get together and have something good to eat at least once a day. That's what human life is all about—enjoying things."

—Julia Child

# SEARED SCALLOPS OVER SPINACH

WE LIKE TO BE able to taste the buttery mildness of the scallops, so instead of complicating the flavors, we keep them simple with lemon juice and mild grapeseed oil. Grapeseed oil has a high smoke point and will get your pan hot, which, along with having very dry scallops, is the trick to getting that perfectly crisp and beautifully browned outside while keeping the inside tender. SERVES 4

1 pound fresh sea scallops

2 teaspoons chopped fresh oregano

2 tablespoons fresh lemon juice (about 1 small lemon)

2 tablespoons grapeseed oil

2 garlic cloves, minced

⅛ cup dry white wine

4 cups fresh spinach

lemon wedges, for serving

sea salt

black pepper

## HOW WE CREATE

Place the scallops on a large plate and pat dry. Season with sea salt, black pepper, oregano, and lemon juice. In a medium skillet, heat the grapeseed oil, and once hot, add the scallops in a single layer. Sear until each side is golden brown and cooked through, 2 ½ to 3 minutes per side. Transfer the scallops to a plate. In the same skillet, add the garlic and wine and cook for 2 to 3 minutes. Then add the spinach and cook until wilted. Serve the scallops on top of the spinach with a lemon wedge on the side.

# PEPPERED SWORDFISH WITH WARM CHIVE-GARLIC SAUCE

SWORDFISH HAS A MILD and sweet flavor, so we like to spice it up by pairing it with a zesty sauce made with whole-grain mustard and lemon juice. SERVES 4

## FOR THE SAUCE

⅓ cup extra-virgin olive oil

5 garlic cloves, minced

3 (3-inch) anchovies, finely chopped

¼ cup chopped fresh chives

1 tablespoon whole-grain mustard

1 tablespoon fresh lemon juice (about ½ small lemon)

1 teaspoon grated lemon zest

¼ teaspoon red pepper flakes

sea salt

black pepper

## FOR THE SWORDFISH

4 (4- to 6-ounce) swordfish steaks

2 tablespoons extra-virgin olive oil, divided

sea salt

black pepper

## HOW WE CREATE

In a small saucepan, warm the olive oil over medium-high heat. Add the garlic, anchovies, chives, and mustard. Let the ingredients begin to heat up for about 1 minute, then stir together. Let cook for 3 minutes (do not let the garlic burn), then add the lemon juice and stir. When the sauce is fully hot, turn off the stove and stir in the lemon zest and red pepper flakes, and season to taste with sea salt and black pepper. Cover with a lid and set aside.

Preheat the oven's broiler.

Place swordfish steaks on a baking pan lightly coated with olive oil and drizzle each steak with ¼ tablespoon of olive oil, then season with black pepper and sea salt. Broil for 3 to 4 minutes on the first side. Remove the baking sheet from the oven and flip the steaks over. Add another ¼ tablespoon olive oil, black pepper, and sea salt to each steak, and broil for another 3 to 4 minutes. If they are lightly brown and the center flakes with a fork, it's time to eat.

Serve each steak topped with an even amount of warm chive-garlic sauce and a lemon wedge.

# LINGUINE AND CLAM SAUCE

LINGUINE AND CLAM SAUCE always reminds me of Christmas Eve. "Feast of the Seven Fishes" is one of my favorite meals of the year and an Italian-American Christmas Eve tradition in which seven seafood dishes comprise a feast to be enjoyed by all. To this day, there are two times each year that I know, without a doubt, I will be having my dad's famous linguine and clam sauce: Christmas Eve and my birthday. Here is his recipe to share with you. —*Nick* SERVES 4

1 pound Linguine Fresh Pasta Dough (page 131)

½ cup extra-virgin olive oil

1 medium red onion, minced

1 large carrot, minced

1 celery stalk, minced

6 garlic cloves, minced

3 fresh bay leaves

2 tablespoons chopped fresh parsley

8 fresh oregano leaves, chopped

½ teaspoon red pepper flakes

1 cup canned San Marzano tomatoes

a pinch of sea salt

4 (3-inch) anchovies, chopped

½ cup dry white wine

25 to 30 little neck clams, cleaned

½ cup freshly grated Parmigiano-Reggiano cheese

## HOW WE CREATE

Prepare the linguine according to the recipe instructions.

In a large saucepan over medium heat, warm the olive oil and sauté the onion, carrot, and celery until tender, 3 to 4 minutes. Add the garlic, bay leaves, parsley, oregano, red pepper flakes, tomatoes, and a pinch of sea salt. Reduce the heat to low and simmer for about 20 minutes, until sauce is nearly smooth. Add the anchovies and white wine and simmer for about 5 minutes. Add the clams and cover with a lid for 8 to 10 minutes, or until the clam shells pop open. Discard any that do not open. Salt again to taste. Add the cooked pasta. Toss in the pan with the Parmigiano-Reggiano.

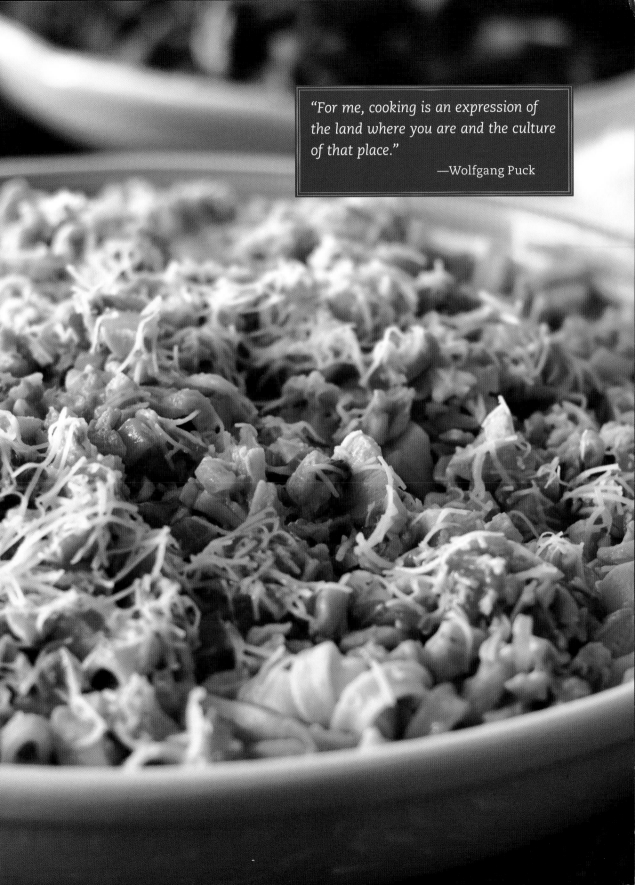

"For me, cooking is an expression of the land where you are and the culture of that place."

—Wolfgang Puck

# BEEF BRACIOLE

AFTER A LONG DAY, my dad and I walk into our home. Italian folk singer Al Martino sings, "I have but one heart, this heart I bring you," in the background, and the smells of Nana's sauce that has been simmering all day put me in an instant state of serenity.

Today when I make this special meal, the house is full of that nostalgic aroma, and I am propelled backward into my adolescence. In my family, this was served as a pasta sauce, but it can be served with just about anything, even as an appetizer. Thank you, Nana. —*Nick* SERVES 6 TO 8

## FOR THE STEAK

½ tablespoon minced garlic

1 tablespoon chopped fresh chives

1 tablespoon chopped fresh parsley

½ tablespoon chopped fresh basil

½ tablespoon chopped fresh oregano

3 tablespoons extra-virgin olive oil

1 tablespoon freshly grated Parmigiano-Reggiano cheese

2 pounds flank steak

sea salt

black pepper

## FOR THE SAUCE

2 (28-ounce) cans San Marzano tomatoes

12 fresh basil leaves, chopped

8 fresh oregano leaves, chopped

3 whole bay leaves

¼ cup extra-virgin olive oil

1 medium red onion, diced

2 celery stalks, minced

1 medium carrot, minced

5 garlic cloves, minced

¼ cup dry red wine

¼ cup freshly grated Parmigiano-Reggiano cheese

sea salt

black pepper

## HOW WE CREATE

To prepare the steak, in a small bowl, mix together the garlic, chives, parsley, basil, oregano, olive oil, and Parmigiano-Reggiano.

Cut the flank steak into 4-inch squares, then lightly season with sea salt. Cover each piece of meat with plastic wrap, then pound with a meat tenderizer, hammer, or other heavy object until each piece is about ¼ inch thick. Unwrap each piece of meat and place them on a flat surface covered with parchment paper. Evenly spread each piece with the garlic mixture and top with a dash of black pepper and sea salt. Then roll up the steak, nice and tight, and close each roll with a toothpick or tie with butcher string. Set aside.

For the sauce, in a large saucepan, add the tomatoes, basil, oregano, bay leaves, sea salt, and black pepper and allow to simmer on very low heat while you cook the meat.

In a large skillet over medium heat, add the olive oil, onion, celery, carrot, and a pinch of sea salt, and sauté for 3 to 4 minutes, until the vegetables begin to soften, stirring occasionally. Then add the steak rolls and sear them on all sides until browned, 2 to 3 minutes on each side. Add the garlic and red wine, and scrape the bottom of the skillet to loosen any browned bits. Add all the ingredients from the skillet into the saucepan and stir. To achieve the best flavor, let simmer, uncovered, for at least 2 hours, but no more than 3 (rolls may fall apart if simmered too long), stirring occasionally. When done, stir in the Parmigiano-Reggiano. Make sure to gently remove the toothpicks or string before serving.

WELLNESS NOTE: Creating this meal is a labor of love. Enjoy your time of cooking and contemplation, of taking in the aromas with a hearty glass of red wine and good company. When you chop, really chop; when you taste, really taste. And when you eat, eat with your entire heart. We recommend making this meal at least once in your life, as the flavors and the preparation seem to sum up...everything.

# WINTER CHICORY WITH PERSIMMONS

WHEN PERSIMMONS START to make their way from the trees to our kitchen, we find any excuse to eat them—often with just a squeeze of lime juice and a sprinkle of cayenne pepper. But on slightly extravagant winter afternoons, we use persimmons to create hearty, nutrient-rich salads like this one. SERVES 4

## FOR THE DRESSING

3 tablespoons fresh lime juice (about 2½ limes)

½ cup extra-virgin olive oil

1 tablespoon chopped fresh thyme

½ teaspoon cayenne pepper

## FOR THE SALAD

7 cups chicory (preferably curly endives)

2 persimmons, sliced (of any variety)

¾ cup chopped pecans

½ cup pomegranate seeds

⅓ cup crumbled blue cheese

sea salt

black pepper

lime slices, for garnish

cayenne pepper, for garnish

## HOW WE CREATE

In a small bowl, make the dressing. Whisk all the ingredients together.

In a large salad bowl, mix the chicory, persimmons, pecans, pomegranate seeds, and blue cheese. Pour the dressing over the salad and toss until evenly coated. Top with sea salt and black pepper. Garnish with a lime slice topped with a sprinkle of cayenne pepper.

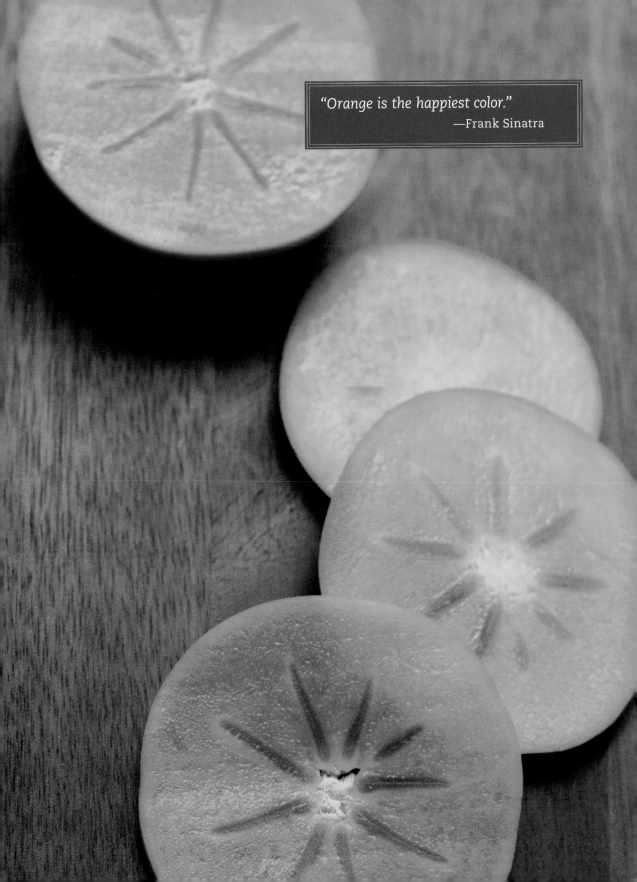

"Orange is the happiest color."
—Frank Sinatra

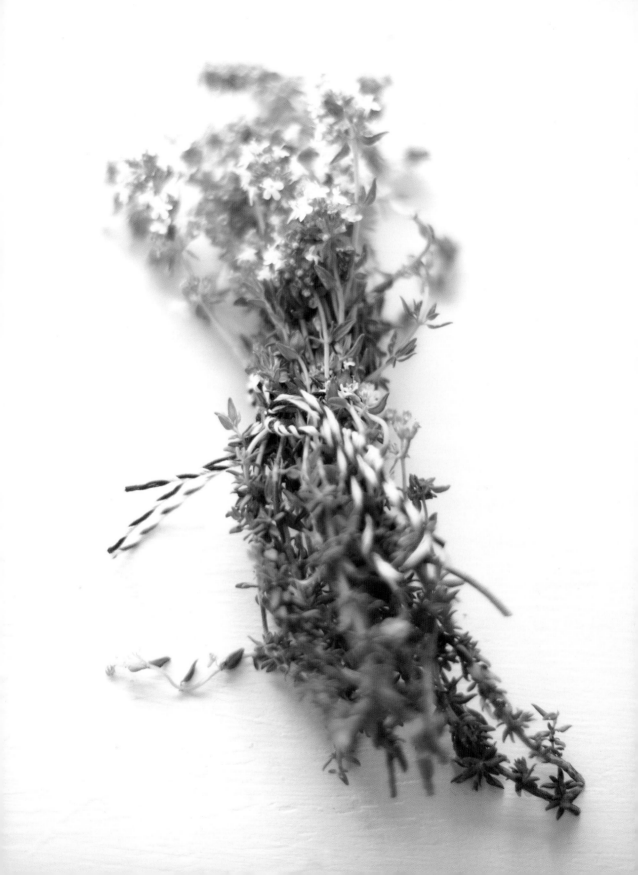

# QUINOA KALE SALAD WITH ROASTED BUTTERNUT SQUASH

OUR FRIENDS OWN a juice bar in Newport Beach called Porrovita, and when our business was just getting started, we'd wake up early to make quinoa kale salads and wraps with homemade tortillas for them to sell. Today, our quinoa salad recipe takes on many different forms, but making it always takes us back to the beginning of *comewecreate*, back to the people who believed in us from the start.  SERVES 4

2 cups cubed butternut squash

½ cup chopped walnuts

½ cup chopped red onion

½ teaspoon ground cinnamon

1 tablespoon chopped thyme

1 teaspoon raw honey

½ cup extra-virgin olive oil, divided

1 cup quinoa

1 bunch kale, stems removed, cut into ½-inch-wide ribbons (about 5 cups)

⅓ cup dried cranberries

1 teaspoon balsamic vinegar

¼ cup shaved Parmigiano-Reggiano cheese (optional)

sea salt

black pepper

## HOW WE CREATE

Preheat the oven to 425°F.

Place the butternut squash, walnuts, and red onion in a large baking dish. Season with sea salt, black pepper, and the cinnamon, thyme, honey, and ¼ cup of the olive oil. Bake for 20 to 25 minutes, until the squash is tender and golden, turning occasionally.

WELLNESS NOTE: Beautiful in shape and color, butternut squash is high in fiber and full of antioxidants and phytonutrients, as well as potassium, folate, and vitamin B6. A shiny skin indicates that the seeded fruit was picked too soon, so go for one with a heavy matte instead.

Meanwhile, in a large pot, bring 2 cups of water to a boil and add the quinoa. Leave the pot uncovered and cook over medium-low heat for about 15 minutes, until the water is absorbed.

In a large bowl, combine the kale, cranberries, balsamic vinegar, and the remaining ¼ cup olive oil and mix. Gently fold in the butternut squash mixture and the quinoa. Top with shaved Parmigiano-Reggiano, if desired. This salad can be served warm or cold.

# ROASTED MEDITERRANEAN BRUSSELS SPROUTS

BRUSSELS SPROUTS are one of our favorites because of they're easy to prepare in a variety of ways. For a more seasonal flavor, we'll bake them with cinnamon, nutmeg, and chopped sweet potatoes. This recipe is more traditionally Mediterranean, but it's simple and filling, and great for throwing together on a cold lazy night after a long day. The feta cheese isn't necessary, but it adds a nice balance of flavors. If you want an extra kick, we suggest adding one chopped red onion and five chopped garlic cloves.  SERVES 4

4 cups trimmed and halved brussels sprouts

1 cup whole artichoke hearts

¾ cup whole, pitted kalamata olives

1½ cups whole baby heirloom tomatoes

2 tablespoons minced fresh rosemary

¼ cup extra-virgin olive oil

4 ounces crumbled feta cheese

sea salt

black pepper

## HOW WE CREATE

Preheat the oven to 400°F.

Combine the brussels sprouts, artichoke hearts, olives, tomatoes, and rosemary in a large baking dish. Drizzle with the olive oil and season with sea salt and pepper. Mix the ingredients well and cook for 30 to 35 minutes, until the brussels sprouts are golden brown and tender. Mix in feta cheese before serving.

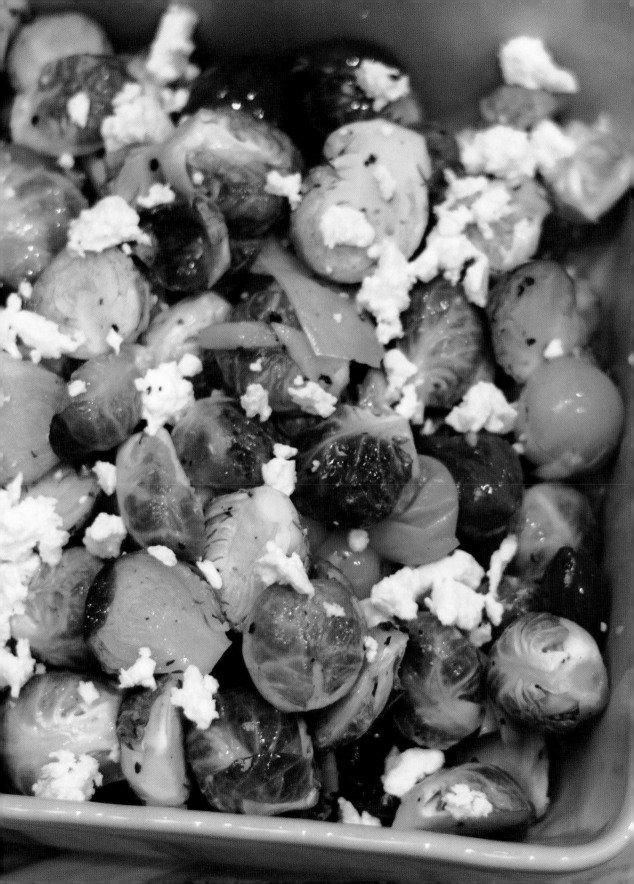

# CHICKEN PICCATA

PICCATA IS A TART DRESSING or sauce (typically citrus) that's used to prepare a meat. Traditional chicken piccata calls for a sauce with heavy butter, but we use extra-virgin olive oil instead. Serve this over a bed of spinach, with a side of asparagus, or with a simple arugula salad for a well-balanced meal. SERVES 4

1 pound boneless, skinless chicken breasts (3 or 4 breasts), pounded ¼ inch thick

sea salt

black pepper

2 eggs, lightly beaten

1 cup white whole wheat flour

¼ cup extra-virgin olive oil

⅓ cup fresh lemon juice (about 2 ½ medium lemons)

1 garlic clove, minced

½ cup chicken stock

¼ cup whole capers, rinsed

1 teaspoon chopped fresh basil

1½ teaspoons chopped fresh dill

3 tablespoons chopped fresh parsley, for garnish

## HOW WE CREATE

Once pounded, season the chicken pieces with sea salt and black pepper. Place the beaten eggs and flour in two separate shallow bowls. Dredge the chicken pieces in the egg and then in the flour and evenly coat, shaking off any excess flour, and place them on a plate.

In a large skillet, bring the olive oil to medium-high heat. Add the chicken and cook for about 3 minutes on each side, or until golden, doing so in batches if needed. Remove and transfer to a plate, covering with foil to keep warm.

Add the lemon juice, garlic, chicken stock, capers, basil, and dill to the skillet and bring to boil. Return the chicken to the skillet and simmer for about 5 minutes. Transfer to a platter. Pour the remaining sauce over the chicken and garnish with parsley.

# DARK CHOCOLATE TANGERINE SLICES

WE FIND A SIMPLE, juicy tangerine to be one of the great pleasures of life. They are the perfect end to a meal, especially topped with a little dark chocolate and a sprinkle of sea salt. MAKES ABOUT 40 PIECES (SERVES 8 TO 10)

8 tangerines (Clementines are best)

3½ to 4 ounces dark chocolate (with at least 70 percent cocoa)

sea salt

## HOW WE CREATE

Line a baking sheet with parchment paper. Peel the tangerines. Using a double boiler, melt the dark chocolate. Dip each tangerine slice halfway into the melted chocolate and place on the baking sheet. Sprinkle with salt and repeat with all the slices. Refrigerate for 10 to 15 minutes, or until the chocolate has hardened.

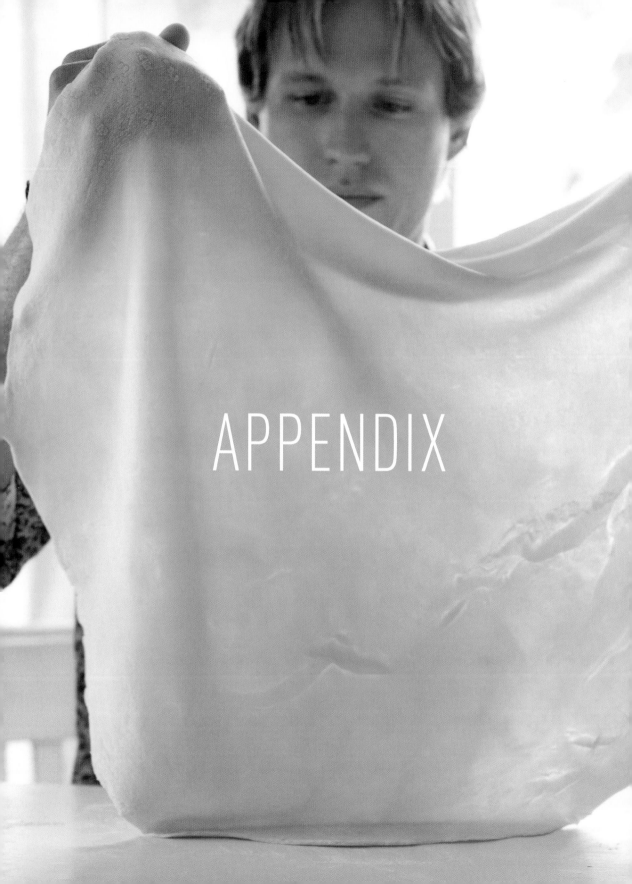

APPENDIX

# FRESH PASTA DOUGH

MAKING YOUR OWN PASTA dough can be so simple, fresh, and fun. The consistency of the noodle is chewier than dried pasta, and we find that we get full faster than we do with store-bought noodles. In the beginning, you'll need to invest some time into the process, but once you get the hang of it, you'll be a pasta-making pro in no time. We find 100 percent whole wheat pasta to be a bit too dense, so when that's what we are in the mood for, we mix equal parts 100 whole wheat and all-purpose flours to soften the overall texture. And, when you're ready to get really creative, try adding some fresh herbs to your pasta, like minced rosemary in your fettuccine or thyme in your farfalle. The possibilities are endless.  MAKES 1 POUND

2 ¼ cups unbleached all-purpose flour,*
plus more as needed

3 eggs, lightly beaten

¼ teaspoon sea salt

1 teaspoon extra-virgin olive oil

2 tablespoons water, plus more as needed

*Note: For whole wheat dough, use equal parts 100 percent whole wheat and all-purpose flour. Double the amount of water, and continue to add water 1 tablespoon at a time, if necessary.

> "Life is a combination of magic and pasta."
> —Federico Fellini

## HOW WE CREATE

On a flat surface, place the flour in a mound and create a large well in the center, adding the eggs, sea salt, and olive oil inside. Using your hands, gently begin to mix ingredients together. Once the flour begins to gather, add the water, 1 tablespoon at a time, and start kneading into a dough. Add more water or flour, as needed. Use the heels of your palms to continue kneading until the dough is elastic and smooth and able to shape into a ball; this could take about 5 minutes. Then cover in plastic wrap and refrigerate for 30 minutes.

Take the dough ball out of the refrigerator and unwrap it. Place it on a lightly floured surface and cut it into 4 equal parts. We do this so it is easier to roll out and to handle (rather than working with one large piece).

One piece at a time, begin to roll out the dough with a flour-dusted rolling pin. Start from the center and roll one direction at a time, making sure to flip the dough over so it does not get stuck on the surface. You might want to sprinkle a pinch of flour onto your work surface a couple times throughout this process. Roll until the dough is about 1/16 inch thick and rectangular in shape.

Until you get used to rolling the dough, it might be a bit thicker and take an additional minute or so to cook. That's okay. Just keep practicing! Like we said, practice makes perfect (or nearly perfect) with pasta. Once you get the hang of it, it's incredibly simple.

Once the pasta sheets are rolled out, sprinkle them with a pinch of flour and let them dry for 5 minutes. Then, if you wish to make the cutting process easier, roll each sheet into a spiral tube and cut to desired shape.

## HAND-CUT PASTA SHAPES

When you are cutting your pasta by hand, as opposed to using a pasta maker or roller, you'll notice that your noodles may not be perfect. Some may be a bit thicker, some thinner, some longer, some shorter. This is okay! Embrace it, as it is a true trademark of entirely *homemade* pasta.

## PAPPARDELLE, TAGLIATELLE, FETTUCCINE, LINGUINE, SPAGHETTI

Use a sharp knife and a ruler (or your free hand) to cut to desired width. In order of widest noodles to thinnest noodles, you will want to cut pappardelle ¾ inch wide, tagliatelle ¼ inch wide, fettuccine ⅙ inch wide, linguine ⅛ inch wide, and spaghetti ¹⁄₁₀ inch wide.

Once your noodles are cut, unroll them (if using spiral tube technique) and place them in a single layer on a flat surface and allow them to dry for about 5 minutes. This will prevent them from sticking to one another while cooking. Place the pasta in boiling water with a sprinkle of sea salt and cook for just 2 to 3 minutes, until the pasta is al dente.

*Note:* Although there are technically different noodle shapes that compliment different sauces, in our recipes and our cooking, we often just ask ourselves, "What kind of noodle sounds good tonight?" It tends to do the trick.

**FARFALLE:** Use a rolling cutter to form pieces that are each 2 inches wide. Unroll the noodles (if using spiral tube technique) then cut the strips 1 inch in length, so you have 2 x 1-inch rectangular pieces. Pinch the middle of each rectangle to form a bow tie shape.

Cook in boiling water with a sprinkle of sea salt for just 2 to 3 minutes, until the pasta is al dente.

**RAVIOLI:** When the ravioli filling is ready and cooled, lay one sheet of pasta dough down on a lightly floured flat surface. Place filling about 2 inches apart on the dough; the amount of filling you use will depend on what size you cut the ravioli, but 1 to 1½ tablespoons is generally standard). Then, place a second sheet of dough on top of the filling. Press on the dough around the mixture to eliminate the air pockets, and cut into shapes using a ravioli cutter, glass cup, or cookie cutter. Pinch the edges to seal.

Cook in boiling water with a sprinkle of salt in batches, so as to give each ravioli enough room. Cook for just 2 to 3 minutes, or until ravioli floats to the top.

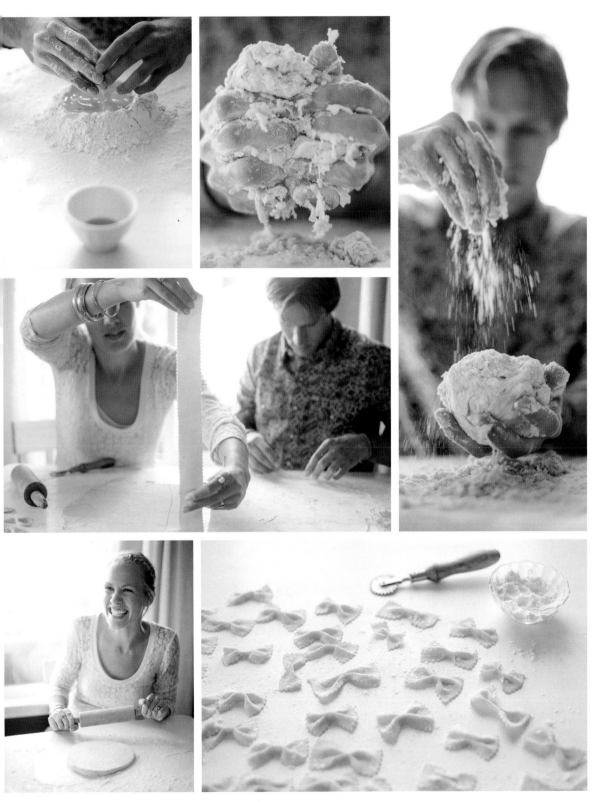

# FRESH PIZZA DOUGH

FOR US, MAKING HOMEMADE PIZZA used to consist of buying the dough from the grocery store and simply adding the ingredients on top of it. Once we began making the dough entirely from scratch, our Friday night pizza dates never tasted so good. Like you can with our fresh pasta, feel free to add herbs to your dough, such as a teaspoon each of minced fresh parsley, oregano, and basil. We hope you too find passion in your pizza making.  MAKES 2 (10-INCH) PIZZAS (SERVES 4)

1 cup lukewarm water

2 teaspoons instant yeast

2 cups unbleached all-purpose flour*

1 teaspoon sea salt

*Note: For whole wheat dough, use equal parts 100 percent whole wheat and all-purpose flour.

## HOW WE CREATE

Preheat the oven to 500°F.

Place the warm water in a large bowl, add the yeast, and stir to dissolve. Let sit for 5 minutes. Add the flour and sea salt. With your hands, mix until dough begins to form. Once it begins to form a loose ball, take the dough out of the bowl and knead with the heels of your hands on a lightly floured surface until the dough becomes stretchy, 4 to 5 minutes or up to 8 minutes. If the dough is sticking to your hands, work more flour in ½ tablespoon at a time.

Form the dough into a ball and place it back into the bowl. Cover the bowl with a clean dish towel and let rise in a warm area for about an hour.

Once the dough has doubled in size, divide the dough in two, place on parchment paper, and roll each piece out with a rolling pin until it becomes about a 10-inch circle. Transfer the pizzas to baking sheets and refer to the specific pizza recipe for further instructions.

# SAMPLE MENUS FOR EVERY-DAYS AND EXTRAORDINARY-DAYS

One of our ultimate favorite things about cooking is menu creation. We love to take the feel of the day and choose our foods intuitively to enhance that feeling. This allows us to get artistic with our eating while simultaneously filling our bodies with the necessary nutrients. We encourage you to use these sample menus as a starting point and let your creativity take you from there.

## SPRING

### SUNDAY SPRINGTIME

Watermelon Gazpacho, page 30

Farfalle Pasta with Arugula, Tomatoes, and Sunflower Seed Pesto, page 36

Lemon-Thyme Sorbet in Lemon Cups, page 48

Grapefruit Mint Prosecco, page 51

### SATURDAY NIGHT ON THE PATIO

Broccoli Pecan Ravioli, page 39

Balsamic-Marinated Portobello Mushrooms, page 45

Caesar Salad with Mesquite Grilled Chicken and Homemade Dressing, page 42

### A SPECIAL OCCASION

Swiss Chard Chardonnay Sauté, page 47

Mediterranean Rice Salad, page 46

Black Peppered Lamb Chops with Mint-Yogurt Sauce, page 34

# SUMMER

SUMMER GATHERING

   Grilled Prosciutto e Melone, page 58

   Caprese Boats, page 54

   Cucumber Salad with Crumbled Feta and Pine Nuts, page 56

   Heirloom Tomato and Kale Pizza with Herb Pizza Dough, page 68

SUNSET BARBECUE

   Eggplant and Kalamata Rolls, page 66

   Wild Salmon on Pecan Wood with Dill-Yogurt Sauce, page 62

   Garlic-Herb Rice, page 70

   Mascarpone and Honey Stuffed Figs with a Balsamic Reduction, page 72

BACKYARD BLISS

   Avocado and Lime Shrimp Cocktail, page 60

   Orange and Fennel Salad with White Wine Citrus Dressing, page 64

   Almond Baked Halibut with Tomato-Caper Sauce, page 65

# AUTUMN

A COLORFUL EVENING

Beet Carpaccio, page 93

Roasted Pumpkin Apple Sage Soup, page 100

Sweet Potato Gnocchi with Honey Crisp Apples, page 90

ROMANCING THE ORDINARY

Baked Lemon and Thyme Mushrooms, page 98

Pear and Prosecco Tilapia, page 95

Garlic-Herb Spaghetti Squash with Lemon, page 88

THE COMFORT OF AUTUMN

Avocado Deviled Eggs, page 78

Zucchini Lasagna, page 85

Simple Sautéed Rapini, page 96

# WINTER

DINNER PARTY DINING

Warm Rosemary Olives, page 106

Winter Chicory with Persimmons, page 122

Linguine and Clam Sauce, page 118

MOMENTS OF THE MEDITERRANEAN

Cioppino, page 110

Roasted Mediterranean Brussels Sprouts, page 126

Seared Scallops over Spinach, page 116

A WARM WINTER

Roasted Fennel and Cauliflower Soup, page 109

Quinoa Kale Salad with Roasted Butternut Squash, page 125

Peppered Swordfish with Warm Chive-Garlic Sauce, page 117

# REFERENCES

Acquista, Angelo, and Laurie Ann Vandermolen. *The Mediterranean Prescription: Meal Plans and Recipes to Help You Stay Slim and Healthy for the Rest of Your Life.* New York: Ballantine, 2006.

Cloutier, Marissa, and Eve Adamson. *The Mediterranean Diet: Lose Weight and Feel Great with One of the World's Healthiest Diets!* New York: Harper Collins, 2001.

Environmental Working Group. "EWG's Shopper's Guide to Pesticides in Produce," April 2014. http://www.ewg.org/foodnews/summary.php.

Jenkins, Nancy Harmon. *The New Mediterranean Diet Cookbook: A Delicious Alternative for Lifelong Health.* New York: Bantam, 2009.

Ozner, Michael. *The Complete Mediterranean Diet: Everything You Need to Know to Lose Weight and Lower Your Risk of Heart Disease.* Dallas: Benbella, 2014.

Raffetto, Meri, and Wendy Jo Peterson. *Mediterranean Diet Cookbook for Dummies.* Hoboken, NJ: John Wiley & Sons, 2012.

# CONVERSIONS

## COMMON CONVERSIONS

| |
|---|
| 1 gallon = 4 quarts = 8 pints = 16 cups = 128 fluid ounces = 3.8 liters |
| 1 quart = 2 pints = 4 cups = 32 ounces = .95 liter |
| 1 pint = 2 cups = 16 ounces = 480 ml |
| 1 cup = 8 ounces = 240 ml |
| ¼ cup = 4 tablespoons = 12 teaspoons = 2 ounces = 60 ml |
| 1 tablespoon = 3 teaspoons = ½ fluid ounce = 15 ml |

# VOLUME CONVERSIONS

| U.S. | U.S. equivalent | Metric |
|---|---|---|
| 1 tablespoon (3 teaspoons) | ½ fluid ounce | 15 milliliters |
| ¼ cup | 2 fluid ounces | 60 milliliters |
| ⅓ cup | 3 fluid ounces | 90 milliliters |
| ½ cup | 4 fluid ounces | 120 milliliters |
| ⅔ cup | 5 fluid ounces | 150 milliliters |
| ¾ cup | 6 fluid ounces | 180 milliliters |
| 1 cup | 8 fluid ounces | 240 milliliters |
| 2 cups | 16 fluid ounces | 480 milliliters |

# TEMPERATURE CONVERSIONS

| Fahrenheit (°F) | Celsius (°C) |
|---|---|
| 200°F | 95°C |
| 225°F | 110°C |
| 250°F | 120°C |
| 275°F | 135°C |
| 300°F | 150°C |
| 325°F | 165°C |
| 350°F | 175°C |
| 375°F | 190°C |
| 400°F | 200°C |
| 425°F | 220°C |
| 450°F | 230°C |
| 475°F | 245°C |

# INDEX

Acquista, Angelo, 13
Adamson, Eve, 12, 13
Alcohol, 22
Almond Baked Halibut with Tomato-Caper
    Sauce, 65
Almond Flour Zucchini-Carrot Breakfast Cake,
    103
Asparagus, Prosciutto, and Mushroom Pizza,
    32–33
Asparagus, raw (wellness note), 33
Autumn recipes, 77–103; sample menus, 137
Avocado (wellness note), 78
Avocado and Lime Shrimp Cocktail, 60–61
Avocado Deviled Eggs, 78
Avocados (wellness note), 61

Baked Lemon and Thyme Mushrooms, 98
Balsamic-Marinated Portobello Mushrooms,
    45
Barley Risotto with Mushroom, Fig, and
    Arugula, 87
Beans, 18–19
Beef. *See* Meat dishes
Beef Braciole, 120–21
Beet Carpaccio, 93
Black Peppered Lamb Chops with Mint-Yogurt
    Sauce, 34–35
Broccoli Pecan Ravioli, 39
Butternut squash (wellness note), 125
Butternut Squash–Pomegranate Hummus, 81

Caesar Dressing, 42–43
Caesar Salad with Mesquite Grilled Chicken
    and Homemade Dressing, 42–43
Caper, Olive, and Sun-Dried Tomato Relish, 40
Caprese Boats, 54
Carbohydrates, 14
Ceviche (wellness note), 67
Cheese, 21–22
Chicken dishes. *See* Poultry dishes

Chicken Piccata, 128
Chicken Sausage Barley Risotto with Rapini
    and Sun-Dried Tomatoes, 114
Chilled Avocado-Cucumber Soup, 55
Chocolate, 22
Cioppino, 110
"Clean Fifteen," 20
Cloutier, Marissa, 12, 13
Condiments, 21
Constipation, 18
Conversions, 138–39
Cooking, and stress, 23
Cucumber Salad with Crumbled Feta and Pine
    Nuts, 56

Dairy products, 21–22
Dark Chocolate Tangerine Slices, 129
Desserts, 48, 71, 72, 128
Dill-Yogurt Sauce, 62
"Dirty Dozen," 20
Dough: pasta, 131–33; pizza, 68, 134
Dressings, 42–43, 64, 122
Drinks, 51

Eggplant and Kalamata Rolls, 66
Eggs, 21
Eggs (wellness note), 78
Exercise, 26

Farfalle Pasta with Arugula, Tomatoes, and
    Sunflower Seed Pesto, 36
Farmers' markets, 25
Fats, 14, 15, 19–20
Fennel (wellness note), 64
Fiber, 18
Fish. *See* Seafood dishes
Food preparation (wellness note), 121
Fruits, 18

Gardening, 24

Garlic-Herb Rice, 70
Garlic-Herb Spaghetti Squash with Lemon, 88
Gelato (wellness note), 71
Grains, 14, 16
Grapefruit juice (wellness note), 51
Grapefruit Mint Prosecco, 51
Grilled Prosciutto e Melone, 58

Heirloom Tomato and Kale Pizza with Herb
    Pizza Dough, 68
Herb gardens, 24
Herb Pizza Dough, 68
Herbs, 21
Honey-Fig Jam, 74
Hummus, 81

Insoluble fiber, 18
Insulin, 18

Jam, 74

Keys, Ancel, 13

Lamb. See Meat dishes
Legumes, 18–19
Lemon-Thyme Sorbet in Lemon Cups, 48
Lemons (wellness note), 48
Lifestyle, 22–27
Linguine and Clam Sauce, 118

Macronutrients, 14
Mascarpone and Honey Stuffed Figs with a
    Balsamic Reduction, 72
Meals, and stress, 23
Measurement conversions, 138–39
Meat, 21
Meat dishes: beef, 120–21; lamb, 34–35; pork,
    32–33, 58
Mediterranean Ceviche, 67
Mediterranean Chicken Stir-Fry, 38
Mediterranean diet, defined, 11–12; dietary
    principles, 13–21; history, 12; lifestyle, 22–27
The Mediterranean Diet, 12, 13
The Mediterranean Prescription, 13
Mediterranean Rice Salad, 46

Menus, sample, 135–37
Micronutrients, 14
Minerals, 14, 16–17
Mint-Carrot Cabbage Wedge, 97
Mint-Yogurt Sauce, 34–35
Monounsaturated fats, 13, 19

Naps, and stress, 23

Olive oil, 20–21
Omega-3 and -6 fatty acids, 19
Orange and Fennel Salad with White Wine
    Citrus Dressing, 64
Organic foods, 25

Pace, and stress, 23
Pasta dishes, 36, 39, 85–86, 88, 90–91, 112–13,
    118; dough, 68, 131–32
Pear and Prosecco Tilapia, 95
Peppered Swordfish with Warm Chive-Garlic
    Sauce, 117
Pesticides, in foods, 20
Pizza, 32–33, 68; dough, 68, 134
Polyunsaturated fats, 19
Pork. See Meat dishes
Portion sizes, 15–16
Positivity, and stress, 24–25
Poultry, 21
Poultry dishes: chicken, 38, 42–43, 94, 114, 128;
    turkey, 112–13
Preparation (wellness note), 121
Processed foods, 13, 24–25
Produce, 14, 17
Proteins, 14; with produce, 17

Quinoa Kale Salad with Roasted Butternut
    Squash, 125

Recipes, 77–129; autumn, 77–103; spring,
    29–51; summer, 53–74; winter, 105–29
Red meat, 21
Red Wine and Garlic Steamed Mussels, 82
Refined grains, 16
Relationships, and stress, 23
Relishes. See Sauces and relishes

Rice dishes, 46, 70, 87, 114
Roasted Butternut Squash, 125
Roasted Fennel and Cauliflower Soup, 109
Roasted Mediterranean Brussels Sprouts, 126
Roasted Pumpkin Apple Sage Soup, 100
Roasted Veggie Tower, 44

Salads, 42–43, 46, 54, 56, 64, 97, 122, 125
Sample menus, 135–37
Saturated fats, 12–13, 19
Sauces and relishes, 34–35, 40, 60–61, 62, 65,
    117, 118, 120, 128
Seafood, 19
Seafood dishes: fish, 40, 62, 65, 67, 95, 110, 117;
    shellfish, 60–61, 82, 110, 116, 118
Seared Scallops over Spinach, 116
Sedentary lifestyle, 26
Serving sizes, 15–16
Shellfish. See Seafood dishes
Simple Sautéed Rapini, 96
Smoothies, 17
Socializing, and stress, 25
Soluble fiber, 18
Sorbet, 48
Soups and stews, 30, 55, 100, 107, 109, 110
Spaghetti and Turkey Meatballs, 112–13
Spearmint-Pistachio Gelato, 71
Spices, 21
Spring recipes, 29–51; sample menus, 135
Stress, reducing, 23–25
Stews. See Soups and stews
Summer recipes, 53–74; sample menus, 136
Sweet Potato Gnocchi with Honey Crisp Apples,
    90–91

Sweet potatoes (wellness note), 91
Sweets, 22
Swiss Chard Chardonnay Sauté, 47

Tomato-Caper Sauce, 65
Tomatoes, heirloom (wellness note), 68
Toxic foods, eliminating, 25–26
Trans fats, 19
Tuna Steaks with Caper, Olive, and Sun-Dried
    Tomato Relish, 40
Turkey dishes. See Poultry dishes
Tuscan Tomato and Cannellini Bean Soup with
    Kale, 107

Vegetables, 16–17; color, 17
Vitamins, 14, 16–17

Warm Chive-Garlic Sauce, 117
Warm Rosemary Olives, 106
Water, 14
Watermelon Gazpacho, 30
White Wine Citrus Dressing, 64
Whole grains, 14, 16
Whole Roasted Apple-Rosemary Chicken, 94
Wild Salmon on Pecan Wood with Dill-Yogurt
    Sauce, 62
Wine, 22
Winter Chicory with Persimmons, 122
Winter recipes, 105–29; sample menus, 137

Yoga, and stress, 23

Zucchini blossoms (wellness note), 44
Zucchini Lasagna, 85–86

# ACKNOWLEDGMENTS

Infinite thanks to the people who follow. You are beautiful.

To Libbey Glass and Angie Kelly, for providing us with a plethora of lovely glassware and tableware. The Sixties Stella still remain to be some of our very favorites, of which we have had many-a-cheers with those we love.

To Todd Porter and Diane Cu, for the bountiful amounts of inspiration you have given us in food, in photo, and in life, for sharing your knowledge and opening your hearts to two kids with big dreams.

To Anthropolgie, TJ Max/Homegoods, Sur La Table, and Williams-Sonoma for the endless prop-spiration. You're a dream to work with.

To the Trader Joe's, Whole Foods, and Sprouts employees of Newport Beach and Tustin and all over the West Coast, really, for providing us with the smiles that fueled these recipes and for giving us a sense of home no matter where we were. And for the wondrous wine deals, of course.

To the family and friends who inspired these creations. We love you immensely.

To Kayla Sampson and Amber Thrane of Dulcet Creative for the deep belly laughs and for shooting the springtime table. And to Meiwen Wang, for photographing the autumn spread and being an overall doll. You are all talented beyond words.

To Keith Riegert and Ulysses Press for reading our first email and taking a chance on us.

To Rea Frey, for being a nutrition magician and for sharing your words and your knowledge.

To all of the designers and editors who have worked to bring this creation to fruition and to Kourtney Joy and the PR team for pushing it forward.

And, of course, to Alice Riegert, our editor, for the back and forths, the honesty, and the ideas and for sitting alongside us on this roller coaster that is a first cookbook. You are truly a gem.

To all of the places we have lived throughout the creation of this book, and to finding our home—which we have come to realize, is nothing more than the meals we share and the memories we make.

And to you, of course, wherever you are, for allowing us into your kitchen and into your lives. We can't wait to see what you create. Make sure to throw a hashtag our way #comewecreate, so we can all collaborate to form a community of inspiration.

# ABOUT THE AUTHORS

**Nick Nigro** and **Bay Ewald** are cofounders of comewecreate, a boutique culinary arts company that focuses on all things imaginative within the realm of food. You can try their unique and healthy menu items (including variations of the Watermelon Gazpacho, Caprese Boats, and Beet Carpaccio from this book) at Avatar Cafe in Long Beach, California. Nick and Bay recently moved from Orange County, California, to Portland, Oregon, where aside from being passionate foodies, they are also in-progress novel writers, creative filmmakers, and devout nature wanderers. Follow their adventures on Instagram @comewecreate or visit their website at www.comewecreate.com.

**Rea Frey** is an award-winning author, nutrition specialist, and International Sports Sciences Association certified trainer. She is the author of *Detox Before You're Expecting: A Cleansing Program to Prepare Your Body for Pregnancy*, *Power Vegan: Plant-Fueled Nutrition for Maximum Health and Fitness*, and *The Cheat Sheet: A Clue-by-Clue Guide to Finding Out If He's Unfaithful*. She lives in Nashville with her husband and daughter.